BROADENING THE DEMENTIA DEBATE

Towards social citizenship

Ruth Bartlett and Deborah O'Connor
with a foreword by Jim Mann

This edition published in Great Britain in 2010 by

The Policy Press
University of Bristol
Fourth Floor
Beacon House
Queen's Road
Bristol BS8 1QU
UK

Tel +44 (0)117 331 4054
Fax +44 (0)117 331 4093
e-mail tpp-info@bristol.ac.uk
www.policypress.co.uk

North American office:
The Policy Press
c/o International Specialized Books Services (ISBS)
920 NE 58th Avenue, Suite 300
Portland, OR 97213-3786, USA
Tel +1 503 287 3093
Fax +1 503 280 8832
e-mail info@isbs.com

© The Policy Press 2010

British Library Cataloguing in Publication Data
A catalogue record for this book is available from the British Library.

Library of Congress Cataloging-in-Publication Data
A catalog record for this book has been requested.

ISBN 978 1 84742 177 7 paperback
ISBN 978 1 84742 178 4 hardcover

Cover design by The Policy Press.
Front cover image kindly supplied by Dez Pain.
Printed and bound in Great Britain by Hobbs, Southampton.

For my daughter Florence, who helps me in more
ways than she knows (RB)

For my mother, Kathleen O'Connor, who has been my role
model and a constant source of support, throughout this
book and my life. (DO)

Contents

List of tables and figures

Tables

Figures

Acknowledgements

This book stemmed from an invitation by Professor Judith Phillips, series editor for the Ageing and the Lifecourse Series, to write about people with dementia. We welcomed the opportunity to extend and apply the ideas we had developed in a previous article (Bartlett and O'Connor, 2007), and for this we are grateful to The Policy Press.

Ideas do not develop in a vacuum. We would like to acknowledge the importance of our discussions with, and support from, our colleagues in our respective units, the Bradford Dementia Group (BDG) and the Centre for Research on Personhood in Dementia (CRPD). We are particularly grateful to Murna Downs, who initially recognised the synergy in our ideas and suggested our writing partnership. Most of all, we are grateful to those individuals with a diagnosis of dementia – people like Lynn Jackson, Jim Mann, Richard Taylor, James McKillop, Edward McLaughlin, Agnes Houston, Heather Roberts – who have shown us how important it is that we as professionals, researchers and general members of society challenge how we understand and respond to dementia.

Funding for any project plays a critical role in the unfolding of ideas. Ruth is especially grateful to the Economic and Social Research Council (ESRC), who funded her PhD study and current research into the experiences of people with dementia who campaign for social change. Without their continued investment and endorsement, the conceptualisations of citizenship presented in this book would not have been possible. Deborah would like to acknowledge the importance of funding through the Canadian Institute on Health Research, which facilitated the development of this international collaboration. Also, the infrastructure support from the Michael Smith Health Research Foundation (MSHRF) was essential for facilitating the development of an interdisciplinary research centre where ideas around personhood and citizenship could be debated and developed.

Series editor's foreword

Judith Phillips

Dementia is an increasingly important issue in policy and practice; yet it receives less research funding than many other areas of ageing, is under-conceptualised, with primarily a psychological or medical approach, and is concerned with care or clinical practice. This timely book seeks to challenge this. It highlights the increasing importance of the study of dementia, challenges our stereotypes, providing more positive associations and gives people with dementia a voice as Jim Mann so eloquently outlines in his foreword. It views people with dementia as active citizens engaged in society and with responsibility and agency in shaping their future. It builds on the work of Tom Kitwood, seeing the person first rather than the 'dementia sufferer', and broadens the debate around personhood to incorporate multidimensional, critical and sociopolitical perspectives. The book uses the concept of social citizenship as a guiding framework and challenges the medicalisation and welfarist approach traditionally seen in policy and practice. Consequently the book provides an invaluable source to all professionals and academics wishing to understand and improve the situation of people with dementia.

The book will bring the latest thinking on dementia with implications for policy and practice and will appeal to an increasingly multidisciplinary audience concerned with the quality of dementia care. In line with other books in the series it stresses the importance of a lifecourse approach, seeing people with dementia in the broader context of their lifecourse and their life cycle.

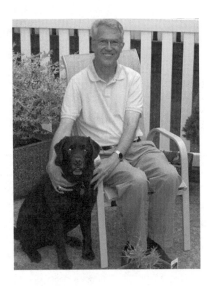

Foreword by Jim Mann

I have become a storyteller. Not with jokes or funny stories, although funny things happen to me a lot. But to tell others about living with Alzheimer's. To tell people my story, my hopes and my intentions and, more importantly my expectations.

Breaking the stereotype of a person with Alzheimer's or other dementia as very elderly and in the final stages is very important to me. And it starts by speaking out, one person at a time.

Like I did to the business acquaintance who sends emails to a broad address list. One day he sent a message that made me think and reflect.

He started his email, 'Even with my failing memory I don't recall …'. I knew he didn't have cognitive impairment and at that particular moment his casual reference to memory loss pushed my buttons. I then knew I needed to be an advocate and to educate. I hit the 'Reply' button and said for the first time since my diagnosis, out loud and with confidence, 'I have Alzheimer's'.

That one incident made me realise that if I don't speak up an opportunity is lost. The stigma continues and so does the lack of understanding about Alzheimer's and related dementias. But more importantly I am lost as a person with Alzheimer's. My concerns and issues get diminished or at best are drowned out. I lose my voice and more importantly the chance to make a difference.

I believe that is called self-advocacy. And engaging in such activity personalises my disease in my terms. I take advantage of my voice to frame the discussion around dementia-related issues and care.

I am a person with dementia. I am also a family member, who has learned a lot from watching and navigating my mother through her dementia journey. I was her advocate before she went into care and then while she was a resident in a care facility.

The lessons learned then and those recently acquired through my own experiences have come together for me and hopefully others like me. I recognise that I have much to teach others. Through my efforts if one doctor or nurse or care aide learns something new and practical about dementia care it's worth it.

It doesn't stop there. The information sharing with the personal voice is vital because there are many links in the chain of those involved in dementia care. I realised that I also needed to try to influence policy makers.

So I wrote a letter. I wanted my government and the minister responsible for advanced education to hear directly some of my concerns about dementia care because, as I wrote, 'front line personnel are key to a successful healthcare system, especially for those residents in care facilities'.

I wrote in part:

> Care aides and nurses do not understand dementia-related residents, bottom line. They have a seeming lack of practical knowledge, which is troublesome because our residents deserve better.'
>
> Their treatment generates frustration from residents, which in turn can result in staff believing the resident is aggressive and needs restraint or some other remedy.
>
> Incidents like a resident with dementia approaching the nurse's station in obvious distress saying she didn't know where her room was and getting in response: "How old are you, dear? Double that and find your room." The poor woman still had no idea where her room was, plus her room number is 99 so that calculation made no sense anyway. On the surface and with someone of sound mind this response is somewhat funny but to a person with dementia it adds to the confusion and is totally unnecessary and unsatisfactory.
>
> There are other incidents that should not be occurring to residents but happen because, in my opinion, there is little if any information during the nurses' and aides' curriculum on the practical knowledge of working with people with dementia.
>
> The fact that I too am a person with Alzheimer's – I was diagnosed at the age of 58, two years ago – makes this perhaps more personal to me. That said, it is because of my diagnosis that I have learned more and am able to offer this assessment to you. What I suggest is not an extraordinary level of education or something beyond what is a fair and reasonable level of care.

I ended the letter with:

> I know it is not lost on you that people with Alzheimer's and related dementias are increasing in number every day, both with earlier

diagnosis and as our baby boomer group ages. Can't we therefore expect a better level of care than I see currently and can't we expect the Government of the day to address this immediately with a pertinent course curriculum?

Only by raising our collective voices can we make a difference in raising awareness among the community-at-large and with medical and care staff. Only by putting a face to the disease will it become personal. And that's how we can make a difference. And that is how we can improve our own environment.

We are not all victims. We have a life worth living. While it may not be the life we would choose it's what we have.

So you know what?

We are going to make it ours. And we're going to make it worthwhile.

We're going to make our mark in the world and be proud of who we are.

And this book is a good step towards making change happen. It raises new questions and shifts the focus away from the way it has always been to a new and sharper image of what it means to be truly 'person-centred'.

This is a positive model that needs to be better understood and valued. Thank you to the authors for acting as change agents.

Jim Mann was diagnosed with Alzheimer's in February 2007. He is now an advocate utilising his experience and expertise in the business and volunteer sectors and as a care partner for his mother who also had the disease. He is active at both the provincial and national level: his many hats including being a board member on the: National Advisory for the Canadian Dementia Knowledge Translation Network (CDKTN); Alzheimer Society of Canada (ASC) Board of Directors and Alzheimer Society of British Columbia (ASBC) Board of Directors. He is also an active member of the Community Advisory Committee of the Centre for Research on Personhood in Dementia (CRPD) located at the University of British Columbia.

Part I
Social citizenship in theory

ONE

Introduction

"I am 46 years old and have the early stages of frontotemporal lobe dementia.... As of now, not many people have decided to 'come out of the closet' so to speak, to tell others their story, to tell people what is wrong them. With a lot of hard work, a wonderful doctor, the passage of time, love from family and friends and other people with dementia, I have for the most part overcome this stigma." (Jackson, 2009)

"I am Richard Taylor, and for nearly a decade I have lived with the diagnosis of dementia, probably of the Alzheimer's type. I have discovered that thinking, speaking, and writing about what it is like for me to live with this condition has become the purpose of my life." (Richard Taylor, PhD, www.richardtaylorphd.com/)

"My name is Terry Pratchett, author of a series of inexplicably successful fantasy books and I have had Alzheimer's now for the past two years plus, in which time I managed to write a couple of bestsellers. I have a rare variant. I don't understand very much about it, but apparently if you are going to have Alzheimer's it's a good one to have. (Terry Pratchett, addressing the Alzheimer's Research Trust Conference in the UK, March 2008, www.terrypratchettbooks.com/)

The theme of World Alzheimer's Day 2007 was: 'No time to lose – people with dementia speak out!'. And people have. After decades of being silenced, marginalised and discriminated against, people with dementia are beginning to use their voice and to speak out about their experiences. Men and women like Richard Taylor, Lynn Jackson, Jim Mann and Terry Pratchett have spoken at major conferences and public events to raise awareness of the discrimination they and other people with dementia face. Others have spoken or written candidly about the impact of dementia on their everyday lives in newsletters, at health committee meetings, through the media and in other public spheres. More still have participated on decision-making boards and taken part in fundraising and consultation events. Importantly, those without dementia are listening: Lynn, Richard and Terry have all been given a standing ovation when they presented their stories at major international conferences.

The call for people with dementia to speak out suggests that this group are now being seen not only as people but also as equal citizens, with the power to influence and bring about social change. Further, as a new generation of people with dementia are willing and able to respond to calls for such action, a new vision is being strengthened and cultural stereotypes of this group as frail, inept and completely incapable are being convincingly challenged. This book is about these new trends and directions and the associated changes in the image, status, role and responsibilities of people with dementia in today's society. It is about the agency, power and social practices of people with dementia. It is about how to recognise, hear and respond to these new trends.

In the influential text *Dementia reconsidered*, Kitwood (1997a) began to paint a new picture of dementia. Rather than seeing dementia in purely clinical terms, as a neurological disease, he gave shape to a more holistic view of dementia in which the person (rather than the disease) came first. This vision raised the status of people with dementia, from 'dementia sufferer' to 'person with dementia', and encouraged us to see individuals with dementia as whole people, rather than 'tragic victims' of a progressive disease.

Since then not only has a new picture of dementia emerged, it has been incorporated into the public policies of forward-thinking governments throughout many parts of the world. For example, many countries, including Australia, Britain, Canada, France, the Netherlands, Norway, and India, have in place or are talking about a National Dementia Strategy in an effort to raise the profile of dementia. While there is still much work to be done in this regard, particularly among the general public and in certain parts of the care sector, the importance of seeing the person first has become a familiar message. Moreover, it has helped to create the climate of opportunities that we see today, in which people with dementia are more prepared and have greater opportunities to speak out. An important question remains, however, and that is: has it taken the picture far enough?

The central argument underpinning this book is that the picture of dementia needs to broaden and continue to evolve once again. It needs to move beyond seeing the individual person as a passive care recipient to seeing the person as an active social agent in the broad context of their lifestyle, lifecourse, social networks and community activities. This book aims to move beyond the conventional focus on welfare recipient that has influenced so many of the discussions about dementia, arguing that this narrow focus fails to take account of other social statuses, entitlements, practices and experiences of people with dementia.

It is designed to support and advance new forms of dialogue and thinking about people with dementia as active citizens. It is primarily about social, political and cultural dynamics, rather than individual clinical or social psychology. It acknowledges the actual and potential contribution of individuals to everyday life in a range of settings and contexts, including, for example, political campaigns, self-advocacy groups, public meetings, conferences and research studies. Moreover, it extends current debate by taking account of the power of people with dementia to combat malignant forces and to contribute to civic life while simultaneously recognising how society may serve to disable rather than enable individuals.

Other literature has focused on the importance of the triadic caring relationship between the person with dementia, professional caregiver and spouse. In this text we assume the importance of this as a given priority, but suggest attention must also be drawn to the other bonds, links and encounters that people may have, such as those with other people with dementia, community groups and mental health networks, voluntary associations, higher education institutions, schools, researchers – even government ministers and heads of state. For example, in March 2009, members of the Scottish Dementia Working Group (SDWG) met with Scotland's First Minister, Alex Salmond MSP, to discuss the ways in which the group had been supported by Comic Relief. One of the members of this group has also met the Queen. Civic relationships like these are rarely discussed in the dementia field and yet they obviously play an important part in a person's life. The core message underpinning the discussions in this book is that the debate about dementia is not just about seeing a person; it is about seeing a person as an active social agent.

An important theme throughout this book is the need to recognise the other social statuses and actions of people with dementia. It refreshes and builds on Kitwood's thesis about seeing the person, not just the disease, by revealing and exploring the myriad of ways in which people with dementia are maintaining and asserting personhood, forming coalitions, claiming rights, becoming politically active, exercising agency, taking control, risks and responsibilities, speaking up for themselves and others, and dealing with the demands of citizenship within the context of having dementia. In particular, the book adds to the priority message about hearing the voices of people with dementia in that it highlights people's political voice – that is, the voice people use to argue for their rights and/ or complain about poor practice – and outlines the ways in which the political voice of people with dementia might be heard and acted on. A goal is to support and open up thinking about the wider experiences and actions of people with dementia and to finally bury the idea that individuals with this condition are necessarily incapable, weak and a burden.

A second core theme underpinning the book is that in order to do this – to reframe how we have understood the capabilities and potential of people with dementia – we need to examine how lived experiences of dementia are entwined, shaped and constrained by broader societal structures and discourses. Thus this book takes an explicitly sociopolitical perspective in an effort to supplement conventional approaches that have prioritised either biomedical or psychosocial factors.

Why the debate must broaden

It has been over a decade since Kitwood and others first began to debate the status of people with dementia, and over a decade since a conceptual framework for understanding and theorising the personhood needs and experiences of people with dementia was first introduced. In that time much has changed. Campaign groups like Dementia Advocacy Support Network International (DASNI) and SDWG – run *by* and for people with dementia – have been set up, challenging public perceptions of people with dementia as excluded, passive, frail and totally incapable. In addition, people with dementia are more likely than ever before to be actively involved in conference proceedings, teaching sessions, research and service evaluation projects, and to be making use of file-sharing websites like 'Flickr' and 'YouTube'. Contemporary networks and forms of communication like these are fundamentally shifting the dementia landscape, raising questions about the currency – or at least completeness – of a conceptual framework developed over a decade ago. This, then, is the first reason for broadening the discussion, to begin to take into account these new trends.

A second reason for broadening the debate is to provide an additional lens for understanding dementia in order to foster a more comprehensive, multifaceted picture. To date the main lenses for understanding people's experiences have been neurological and/or psychosocial. Problems with sole reliance on a neurological lens have already been widely debated and these critiques are not repeated in this book. However, the limitations of a psychosocial lens have received less attention. This has led to certain processes and problems being seen but not others. For example, people's experiences of dementia have largely been analysed using more psychologically oriented constructs such as 'awareness', identity' and 'coping strategies' and the sociopolitical aspects of people's lives have largely been ignored. As a result, issues facing men and women with dementia beyond the care setting, including those related to socioeconomic status, discriminatory attitudes, public transport and work, have not been given the attention they merit. This book brings to the fore a more sociopolitical understanding of the situation of people with dementia and seeks to provoke debate about people's status as citizens. Psychosocial perspectives on dementia are not ignored or relegated as unimportant; on the contrary our intention is to build on existing knowledge in order to pave the way for a richer, more complex, understanding of the changing situation and statuses of people with dementia.

Related to the above, a third reason for broadening the debate is to raise awareness of the heterogeneity of people with dementia. While the idea of treating people as individuals is widely promoted in the dementia field, there is a tendency, conceptually at least, to homogenise people's experiences of dementia – to see everybody in the same terms. It is rare in scholarly debate, for instance, to hear discussions about younger men with Lewy Body Dementia, or to find analysis of the situation facing single older women with dementia on a low income. Indeed, there is very little gendered or socioeconomic analysis of people's experiences of dementia. With few exceptions, social location, with its attendant privilege and disadvantage, is rarely incorporated into discussion. This is perhaps surprising given that different groups of people will undoubtedly have very different experiences of dementia.

It is assumed, for example, that everyone will experience stigma and discrimination equally and continually; the possibility that responses may be far more varied than this is often overlooked. Lynn Jackson, for instance, found it possible to overcome the stigma, and the chair of SDWG said at the closing ceremony of the *Journal of Dementia Care* Congress in Harrogate 2009, "my dementia is wonderful", suggesting that stigma is not always a problem for him. Consistent with this, Hulko (2009) documented very different interpretations of dementia between those who were multiply disadvantaged and those who had historically been more privileged. The tendency to emphasise the collective experiences of people with a disability as an oppressed and disadvantaged group in society, while helpful in terms of raising awareness and galvanising resources, can also be counterproductive in that it over-simplifies people's experiences (Priestley, 2004).

Moreover, a person's experience of dementia will be different depending on where the person is in their life cycle. This is because 'processes of identification (continue to) unfold for individuals as they age' (Hockey and James, 2003, p 20). Lynn Jackson, for instance, was in her forties (mid-life) when she was diagnosed with frontotemporal lobe dementia, working in a 'dream job' in Mexico City; however, when the dementia caused Lynn to swear excessively at work, she was forced to take an abrupt career/lifestyle change (Jackson, 2009). Many others will be in their eighties (later-life) when they are diagnosed with dementia, and may have different priorities and lifestyle changes to make. The point is, 'disability carries a different significance for people of different ages and at different stages of their life course' (Priestley, 2004, p 94). Hence, the debate must broaden and take account of lifecourse differences.

In summary, there are three main reasons why the debate about dementia must be extended. First, a lens that is more consistent with the current reality of many people with dementia as active, engaged and socially contributing to society is needed. In short, a more hopeful lens is needed. Second, a more complex, comprehensive perspective is needed – one that moves beyond individualised discourses about disease and adaptation in order to develop a multidimensional approach to change. Third, a more critical perspective is needed in order to challenge the assumed homogeneity of dementia experiences and to recognise how positions of social advantage and disadvantage related to social location and stage of life influence day-to-day experiences.

Drawing on critical perspectives to broaden debate

In this book a consciously critical perspective is taken in order to broaden the debate. The book constitutes a timely contribution to the Ageing and the Lifecourse Series in that it brings together disparate areas of literature to provide a thorough and critical reappraisal of the situations of people with dementia. It crosses traditional subject boundaries and draws on a wide range of theories and disciplines – including critical gerontology, disability studies, feminism and critical psychiatry – to debate key issues. In order to situate our perspective, a brief explanation of what is meant by a critical perspective from each of these stances is provided below. The intent is to identify how each has been drawn on to inform our thinking.

Critical gerontology provides an umbrella for pulling together the ideas presented in this book. From a gerontological stance, a critical perspective is one that 'goes beyond everyday appearances and the unreflective acceptance of established positions' (Estes et al, 2003, p 3). On this basis we must always question why something is the way that it is, even if the 'usual way' is accepted by everyone as common practice. For example, proposing to extend ideas related to person-centred dementia care, including the emphasis on 'personhood', is to question a position which to date has been deemed sacrosanct. The point is not to critique for the sake of critiquing but rather to improve the domain of practice on which established norms and ways of thinking are based. This is done, at least in part, by attending to what is excluded. In this book, an important part of this process is the examination of structural inequalities, questioning why such inequalities, especially those related to age, gender, 'race', class, disability and sexuality, are so often ignored. Drawing on this perspective, one of the aims of this book is to bring to the fore a critical analysis of how structural issues influence the day-to-day experiences of living with dementia.

Disability studies offers one lens for facilitating this analysis. Within this field, a critical perspective is one that emphasises and examines the problems in society. The focus of debate is not the individual and their impairment but rather societal issues, such as physical and attitudinal barriers, created by the majority non-disabled population, that limit people's full participation in everyday life. Advocates of this stance argue for the removal of barriers and the promotion of the individual and collective empowerment of people with disabilities (Barnes et al, 1999). Key characteristics of this perspective are that it: (a) couches any discussions of the experiences of people with disabilities within an environmental and sociocultural context; and (b) highlights the disabling consequences of a society organised around the needs of a non-disabled majority.

While this offers a useful lens, some disabilities scholars have been critiqued for being too one-sided and negating the barriers caused by impairment. This is not the intention of this book. Rather, we draw on the ideas of second wave disability theorists who have argued that the way forward is to fully integrate the experience of impairment with the experience of disability (see, for example, Corker, 1999; Crow, 1996; French, 1993). Our intent in using critical disability theory as a lens is to take into account social barriers but also to recognise the impact of the neurodegenerative changes that are happening to a person with dementia. Terry Pratchett, for example, clearly articulates the challenge that visuoperceptual changes have been for him. Clearly the experience and impact of neurological impairment cannot and should not be ignored, particularly when talking about citizenship practices, but they must be understood within the context of social processes and structures.

Feminism offers an additional critical lens that has provided essential guidance in developing the ideas of this book. This body of literature has grappled with issues related to social positioning and intersectionality, and provides a language for understanding stigma and power within a context of ageism, disability, gender and socioeconomic disadvantage – to name a few of the potential sites of oppression that commonly overlap for those with dementia. Additionally, since the early 1980s, feminist theory has been developing a feminist ethics of care that is particularly pertinent to dementia studies. A feminist ethics draws attention to the problematics associated with how care has been conceptualised including attacking the dichotomy between giving and receiving care, and theorising a more dynamic, relational understanding. Finally, feminist research methods provide important inroads for employing approaches to knowledge development that both address issues of power in the research process and offer analytic strategies for making the links between lived experiences and broader societal structures and systems.

The fourth critical school of thought that informs the ideas of this book is *critical psychiatry*. Critical psychiatry can be described as a movement or critique against traditional mental health services, and assumptions about the experiences of people with mental health conditions. Based on the work of French philosopher Michel Foucault, specifically his text *Madness and civilization* (1988), critical psychiatry takes as its starting point the idea that psychiatric services can do more harm than good. A critical perspective from this stance is one that explores the 'relationship between psychiatry, social exclusion and coercion', particularly the 'complex issues surrounding diagnosis and framing, as well as power and priorities' (Bracken and Thomas, 2005, p 14). Debates about the medicalisation of dementia can be seen as directly or indirectly coming from this perspective (see, for example, Harding and Palfry, 1997; Kitwood, 1997a; Bond, 1992). In this book this perspective is drawn on to help make sense of the meaning and value of citizenship.

Combined, these critical perspectives form a basis from which to facilitate a critical perspective in this book that has the following assumptions:

- Disabling experiences must be contextualised within a broader sociopolitical context to be fully understood and changed.
- Those with dementia have an important collective experience, as a group who have been marginalised and stigmatised. However, each person also has unique responses that may be grounded in past and present lifecourse experiences.
- The diverse social positions that people occupy work to advantage and/or disadvantage some more than others. Thus, our intention is to highlight not only the diversity of people's journeys through the lifecourse but also to reveal how people's experiences, particularly of oppression and discrimination, may be attributable to factors other than dementia.

Problem of status

According to the philosopher Karl Popper (1999), human beings are continually creating ideas to resolve problems. Over the past few years a vast range of ideas have been proposed and adopted to resolve problems facing people with dementia.

For example, the idea of person-centred care has been advocated to address the problems associated with failing to see the person behind the dementia diagnosis; relationship-centred care is another attempt to respond to the same problem that draws attentions to relational contexts. Undoubtedly, other ideas will form as our desire to resolve what is an intractable problem continues to grow, and as new solutions render visible new issues.

From our perspective, an essential problem underlying the quality of recognition and treatment afforded to people with dementia, which remains unresolved in dementia studies, is the problem of status, specifically, the lack of social status and regard given to people who are diagnosed with dementia. We are not the first to identify this as an issue. In this book we recognise and welcome the work that has been done to address this problem, particularly by organisations such as the World Health Organization, Alzheimer's Disease International and Alzheimer's societies. However, while inroads are being made, the status of people with dementia, especially those with a dementia that is not Alzheimer's disease, or those from an already marginalised position related to say, another disability, ethnicity or social class, remains extremely low. This is perhaps best evidenced by the fact that most social research focuses on the experiences of white, middle-aged people with dementia and their spouses (Hulko, 2009). One of the aims of this book then, is to identify and generate new ideas and language to help resolve the problem of status.

This book adds to and builds on previous work about the status of people with dementia. In particular, we examine work on the concept of personhood. The personhood lens has done much to raise the profile of people with dementia. It has provided a framework and language for raising consciousness about the status of people with dementia as people, intrinsically worthy of respect, and shifted understanding of dementia from a 'technical (medical) framework' to a humanistic perspective (Kitwood, 1993, p 100). The lens of personhood has arguably become one of the most influential for dementia practice and research in the last decade. However, while the strengths of personhood are widely recognised, the limitations of this lens have been less well understood, particularly in respect to how the concept affects the status of people with dementia. In Chapter Two this book reviews the contribution a focus on personhood has made to dementia practice and research, while also examining the boundaries of personhood for tackling the problem of status.

Our book is based on the belief that greater consideration must be given to the status and positioning of people with dementia as more than welfare recipients. To date, the field has tended to accept unreflectively the primary status of 'welfare recipient' for all people with dementia. Consequently, other social statuses, such as employee, carer, consumer of culture, family member, friend, voter, volunteer, educator – to name but a few – have been overlooked. In this book we reflect on the positioning of people with dementia as welfare recipients and in so doing highlight one of the main problems associated with this process and status, which is that it tends to render people passive, in need and on the same trajectory. We draw on previous work on positioning and argue for the repositioning of people with dementia as active social agents, not simply as welfare recipients.

One of the aims of the book is to re-emphasise the importance of attending to the use of language as a means for tackling the problem of status. Language is an important focus for the book as it is often this that renders people with a disability as docile, unproductive or disempowered (Hughes and Paterson, 1997). For example, expressions such as 'dementia sufferer', 'totally impaired' and 'lacking in insight' – labels frequently used in relation to people with dementia – imply that all people with dementia are always in a constant state of distress, confusion or inarticulateness. Patently people are not. Our intention is to show how inaccurate and unhelpful certain phrases and dialogue about people with dementia can be. We focus on words and linguistic practices which silence people with dementia, and lead them, like people with other disabilities, to be 'excluded from responsibility' and thus afforded very little opportunity to demonstrate or express how socially competent they are (Paterson and Hughes, 1999, p 606). Our discussion builds on work on the 'dialectics of dementia' (Kitwood, 1990) and seeks to provide and encourage more positive and equitable ways of talking and thinking about people with dementia.

As well as focusing on actual words and phrases we examine the general notion of 'dementia care'. In particular, we highlight and explore how terms and expressions such as 'care' and 'need', which derive from medical discourse, have come to dominate the debate in dementia studies and further position people with dementia as welfare recipients. Our discussions draw on work in cognate disciplines where the ideology of care and caring is a contested one and the positioning of people as passive recipients of care is problematic. For example, from a disability perspective, being cared for can be stressful for a person with a disability, as that person may not want, or have a say in, the care they receive (Oliver, 1996). Similarly, it can be experienced as oppressive if too much emphasis is placed on 'cure', and providing pharmacological and other medical treatments (Makin, 1995; Marks, 1999). While there has been some debate within dementia studies about the 'caring culture' and the oppressive effects it can have on an individual (see for example, Kitwood, 1997a; Rundqvist and Severinsson, 1999; Martin and Younger, 2000), there has been little analysis of this matter from a sociopolitical perspective and in relation to the problem of status or discrimination.

A further reason for problematising the status of a person with dementia as welfare recipient is because people with memory problems desire, and are entitled to, more than just 'care'. For example, enforcement of human rights and opportunities related to continued employment may be more important to some; others may be more concerned about better access to public transport, particularly when they may need to give up driving; still others may feel strongly about continuing to exercise their right to vote and/or wish to remain active participants within their local community for as long as possible; and others, like members of the SDWG, clearly value the chance to join forces and campaign. Obviously the wider entitlements of people with dementia will often become intertwined with care needs, particularly if that person is in a long-term care setting, and it is not always possible, or indeed desirable, to distinguish between them. The point this book makes is not that we should necessarily distinguish between different types of need, but that it is far too easy to overlook certain ones, like economic and political needs, if 'welfare recipient' is assumed to be the sole status. The aim of this book, therefore, is to centralise and debate the social and political aspects of people's lives and to analyse care needs in the wider context of the lifecourse.

Towards social citizenship

In this book the concept of social citizenship is drawn on to provide a fresh way of thinking about the status of people with dementia. In related disciplines, including social gerontology, critical psychiatry and disability studies, a citizenship lens is used to promote the status of discriminated groups of people as equal citizens, with similar entitlements and rights to everyone else. These disciplines use citizenship to understand and expose discrimination against marginalised groups such as children and people with physical disabilities, and to reframe and politicise understanding of the experiences of people with mental health conditions (Mind, 1999; Sayce, 2000; Bracken and Thomas, 2005). The scope of this social citizenship lens is wide-ranging and goes beyond care issues to include discrimination in the workplace and communities generally.

Within the field of dementia studies, the concept of citizenship is already beginning to emerge as vital. At the practice level, more and more individuals and organisations, including people with dementia themselves, are talking about the importance of seeing people with dementia as equal citizens with rights and sometimes responsibilities. For example, the first conference of the Dementia Services Development Centre in Northern Ireland was based on the theme of citizenship, and Stephen Judd, Chief Executive of Hammond Care in Australia, used that theme in his keynote address to delegates to stress the importance of belonging for people with dementia.

However, while the concept is increasingly used in dementia discourse, what citizenship actually means in relation to individuals with dementia, particularly those who are severely cognitively impaired, remains unclear and open to interpretation. With its dual focus on rights and responsibilities, this is a concept that requires further fleshing out, in order to examine and develop its usefulness within dementia studies.

Thus, while the need to promote citizenship, as well as personhood, is beginning to be recognised within the dementia care literature (Bond et al, 2004; Cantley and Bowes, 2004; Graham, 2004; Innes et al, 2004), what it means to be a citizen, and how that differs from being a person, is not only under contention generally (Bickel, 1975; Heater, 1999) but also, and more critically, remains under-theorised within dementia practice and research (Bartlett and O'Connor, 2007). Our intention is to contextualise and make the concept of citizenship meaningful to dementia studies and to recast ideas about rights, responsibilities and participation in a way that is relevant and useful.

Recognising the impact of impairment and value of scientific research

In broadening the dementia debate towards social citizenship it is important not to lose sight of the centrality of impairment in people's lives. Being cognitively impaired is a formidable 'mental obstacle' (Walker, 1999) that, as this book will show, creates particular issues when relating the concept of citizenship to people with dementia. Thinking more broadly about the experiences of people with dementia allows for deeper insights into how individuals experience and manage this condition. Moreover, it means people's experiences of dementia are understood in the context of their lifecourse, as opposed to the disease process. It examines in detail the capacity of people with dementia to make a positive and active contribution to everyday life and to negotiate the lifecourse, while recognising the impact of cognitive impairment on a person's ability to do so.

While not the focus of this book, it is important to acknowledge the role of scientific medical research in the dementia field, particularly as advances in molecular biology mean that disease modification (as well as symptom management) is now becoming a real possibility (Holmes and Wilkinson, 2000). Efforts to find a cure and to better understand the pathology of cognitive impairment have led to the establishment of scientific research institutes throughout the world, and biomedically focused research receives the vast amount of research funding going towards dementia research.

However, while scientific work on the aetiology and pathology of dementia is obviously extremely important, there is a danger when too much emphasis and hope is placed on clinical trials and the goal of 'finding a cure' that issues related to quality of life may be overlooked and those people currently experiencing dementia may be left to suffer in silence. Moreover, if our treatment of dementia is seen as a sign of greater societal problems – for example, tendencies to separate mind and body, and to prioritise thinking (cognition) over other ways of being – then medical advancement around abolishing dementia is not the answer. This is not to diminish the importance of a cure: it is important to remember that a delay in the progression of the condition by just five years would halve the disease prevalence (Holmes and Wilkinson, 2000, p 193). Rather, it is to highlight that a focus purely on cure is not enough.

Contribution and structure of the book

The central purpose of this book is first to propose a conceptual framework for understanding the situation of people with dementia that is fresh, dynamic and contextualised, and then examine how this might be used in practice. As already implied, the needs of people with dementia have invariably been seen as psychological in nature and related to a person's experience of either having dementia or being a dementia care recipient. With few exceptions the broader experiences and entitlements of people with dementia *as citizens* are rarely discussed or even considered. The idea that people with dementia are citizens has long been recognised (King's Fund Centre, 1986) and the importance of treating a person with dementia as an active agent has been voiced (Kitwood, 1997b). Clearly, the field must have a conceptual framework that supports and fosters understanding of the full spectrum of the dementia experience.

The purpose of this book is to begin to develop this framework, building on previous work and recognising and integrating the concepts of personhood and citizenship. The framework should be used to help advance thinking about people with dementia as active agents and to examine a range of practices, including case-based work and social research involving people with dementia. The purpose of providing a more integrated conceptual framework – apart from the fact that the field does not have a substantive conceptual framework on which to draw – is that it immediately expands the agenda and helps us to think more broadly about the situation of people with dementia within and beyond care settings.

Extending the conceptual framework is intended to provoke debate and to inspire and equip readers to see and treat people with dementia as not only 'service users' but as equal citizens with interests, concerns and support networks outside of the dementia care setting. This book is not primarily about how to care for people with dementia – there are plenty of other excellent texts on that subject (see, for example, Downs and Bowers, 2008) – but how to think about, relate to and increase the capacity of people with dementia and the community in which they live. Fundamentally, it is about seeing a broader picture.

The book is organised into three parts. Part I introduces a conceptual framework for broadening debate towards social citizenship. It identifies and explains in detail the conceptual features of the framework. Chapter Two sets the context for broadening the debate. It describes and explores key moments in the dementia debate and argues for the injection of a more dynamic and sociopolitical way of thinking and practising. Chapter Three focuses on the concept of citizenship. It reviews and summarises the literature on citizenship and clarifies the meaning, key elements and relevance of this concept in relation to people with dementia. It explains how the concept differs from personhood and discusses its meaning from a range of theoretical perspectives.

Part II applies the conceptual framework in relation to different areas of practice. Chapter Four applies the framework to reflexive practices and examines the implications of thinking and talking about dementia in a more sociopolitical way. Reflecting our understanding of the importance of language for constructing reality, this chapter draws on social constructionism to offer a lens for interrogating the values, beliefs and assumptions we are drawing on to make sense of our interactions with people with dementia. Ways of consciously using language – both written and spoken – to reconstruct a different way of understanding are discussed.

Chapter Five applies the broader conceptual base to social and health care practices. We begin with the premise that most practice is case-based but suggest that the tendency to dichotomise between micro level practice and a more macro level orientation is problematic. To this end, we identify four principles for practice that operationalise the ideas underpinning a critical social citizenship approach to practice and offer strategies that are particularly congruent with these principles.

The notion of 'practice' is extended further in Chapter Six, where the focus is on using and doing research that is both conceptually and methodologically congruent with ideas associated with social citizenship. We build on the notion that we must 'EXPECT' that people with dementia can and should be more involved in the production of knowledge, and use this as an organising framework. This framework suggests actions to be considered for developing a research approach grounded in ideas of social citizenship. These include: re-evaluating what counts as data or 'evidence'; expanding the existing research agenda; using participatory methodologies which address power dynamics and creatively exploring alternative ways of generating data and insights; developing a more sophisticated consideration of ethical issues; employing critical analytic strategies that facilitate the linking of personal experiences and broader societal influences and practices; and finally, finding ways to ensure that research is used and useable.

The third and final part of the book combines theory and practice and pulls together the three themes that are developed in this book. These are: the importance of bringing a sociopolitical perspective to the fore; the relevance of a social citizenship lens for elevating status and recognition of rights of people with dementia; and the importance of seeing beyond the care focus in dementia studies. We recognise that this discussion is just the beginning, and identify questions and ways for moving the debate further.

TWO

Setting the context for broadening the debate

Introduction

For the past 30 years the Western world has seen the evolution of our understanding of dementia emerge through three relatively distinct paradigm shifts or 'moments'. In the first moment, the condition was considered a fairly predictable sign of normal ageing, and hence was largely unremarkable and invisible. For example, in 1982, one of the authors (DO) recollects reading the physician-provided medical diagnosis for an 82-year-old woman with severe cognitive impairment preparing for a move into a care home; it read 'old woman living with old man'. What is somewhat astounding retrospectively is that throughout the discussion about the suitability of this woman to enter this care facility, no one on the seven-person admission committee – composed of health and social care professionals including another physician – challenged this 'diagnosis' (although it was treated humorously). While this may represent an extreme situation, the point remains that relegating problematic cognitive deterioration of an older family member to the expectable realm of 'senility', or simply the ageing process, was not unusual.

The second moment arguably began to dominate by the early 1980s, when the unquestioning acceptance of deteriorating cognitive functioning as a sign of normal ageing was increasingly challenged and relabelled as a biomedical condition; in particular, the recognition that Alzheimer's disease was not simply a disease of younger adults heralded an increasingly biomedical era. This understanding of dementia as a neurodegenerative disorder, characterised by symptoms that included declining memory, insight, judgement and ability to communicate, became the dominant lens within Western culture for understanding many conditions associated with deteriorating cognition in older adults. Using the language of 'dementia', this lens assumes a trajectory of irrevocable decline related to neuropathological changes, and predicts that over time the person with dementia will become progressively more dependent on others for all aspects of his or her care.

The medicalisation of dementia has had important benefits. Perhaps most significantly, it has generated scientific interest and research, which has led to more refined diagnostic practices, including increased precision around earlier diagnosis and prognosis. For example, a whole new category of pre-dementia 'diagnosis', including cognitive impairment, no diagnosis (CIND) or mild cognitive impairment (MCI), is now based on the assumption that we have sufficient understanding of normal and abnormal brain changes to achieve earlier, accurate diagnosis. Moreover, biomedicalisation has led to the development of medications for slowing the progression of some of the dementia disorders.

There have also been social benefits associated with the biomedicalisation of cognitive decline. In particular, obtaining a diagnosis has been useful in assisting family members to access some services and benefits, and to cope more effectively with their relative's deterioration. This is because a diagnosis allows family members to externalise the cause of problematic behaviours – "it's not him/her, it is the dementia" – and better understand what is happening and how to handle it. Furthermore, the process of medicalising dementia has indirectly led to clearer recognition of the family's role in providing care, ensuring that their efforts are both more visible and better supported.

However, according primacy to the biomedical lens for understanding dementia has also had unintended negative consequences. First, with the focus on the 'disease' there is a tendency to negate the person behind the disease; they are relegated to the status of 'the demented' or 'dementia sufferer' and viewed as 'care receivers' rather than as a 'full' person. As we will discuss later, it is becoming increasingly clear that this is both an inaccurate picture and highly problematic. Second, evidence is accumulating to suggest that neurodegenerative changes alone do not always adequately account for the trajectory of the dementia path. There is no doubt that changes in the brain do matter, but separating neuropathology out as the only relevant factor is increasingly challenged as overly simplistic in terms of its explanatory power. Finally, the medical model has been strongly critiqued for its undue focus on deficits and therapeutic nihilism – the person with the disease is defined only by loss and what they *cannot* do.

Responding to the limitations associated with this dominant biomedical paradigm, a third moment began to emerge in the early 1990s based on a more humanistic or psychosocial approach. Arguably, this new understanding has been dominated by attention to personhood. This chapter will examine this third 'moment', highlighting the strengths of this approach but also drawing attention to the limitations. It is argued that the emergence of a fourth moment has now begun – that of a more dynamic, contextualised account of the dementia experience. As a means of moving forward in this moment – and establishing the context for the relevance of social citizenship as an emerging core concept in it – this chapter will conclude by outlining a multidimensional conceptual framework for considering dementia in a way that explicitly draws in a more sociopolitical perspective.

Personhood

Personhood is a contested concept that has generated enthusiastic debate among scholars for centuries. The idea dates back to the Enlightenment and the philosophies of René Descartes (1596-1650) and John Locke (1632-1704) on what it means to be a person. Reflecting its logical empiricist roots, traditional views of personhood focus largely on cognitive abilities, such as consciousness, rationality, intentionality, memory, reciprocity and capacity to communicate (Harrison, 1993).To be a person, it is assumed that you must be capable of rational thinking and memory. Because dementia is associated with a progressive decline in these cognitive functions, the disease has historically been assumed to strip the individual of their personhood status, leading to a 'loss of self' (Cohen and Eisdorfer, 1986; Herskovits, 1995).

Beginning in the late 1980s, the notion of 'personhood' was reconceptualised and introduced into the dementia literature as a critical component of the dementia experience. Challenging traditional understandings that linked it solely to cognitive functioning, personhood was revisioned as socially constructed by and within a person's interactional environment. Tom Kitwood, perhaps one of the most recognised pioneers of this approach, offered the now oft-quoted definition of personhood as 'a standing or status that is bestowed upon one human being by others in the context of particular social relationships and institutional arrangements. It implies recognition, respect and trust' (Kitwood, 1997b, p 7). He challenged that personhood was a property of the individual, suggesting instead that relationship comes first, and with it, inter-subjectivity (Baldwin and Capstick, 2007, p 136). Kitwood stressed the influence of interpersonal relations as an essential aspect for understanding the dementia experience, theorising that at least some of the deterioration seen in people with dementia was caused not by the diseased brain itself, but rather by how the person was treated, which resulted in his or her subsequent loss of personhood. Others, both in the UK and elsewhere, developed compatible ways for conceptualising the dementia experience as relational and not simply cognitive (see, for example, Sabat and Harre, 1992; Cheston and Bender, 1999; Sabat, 2001; Woods, 2001; Davis, 2004).

At a broad level, attention to personhood in the dementia care literature explicitly displaces the biomedical model as the only approach for understanding dementia. Rather than assuming a trajectory of irrevocable decline related to neurodegenerative changes, this perspective recognises that performance, behaviour and quality of life are not solely determined by neuropathology but also by personal histories, interactions with others and by how people are perceived within their social context (O'Connor et al, 2007). Growing evidence supports the importance of this broadening vision by highlighting the inconsistencies between neuropathology and actual behaviour (see, for example, Franssen and Reisberg, 1997; Mitnitski et al, 1999; MRC-CFAS, 2001).

At a more specific level, a focus on personhood in dementia can be credited with developing dementia practice and research in three critical ways. First, this lens has promoted a more holistic – and hopeful – understanding of dementia. Kitwood (1997a) and others clearly accorded primacy to the interpersonal environment for helping to shape the dementia experience; the linear link between personal experience of deterioration and organic changes is challenged and someone's interactions with their world is recognised as having the potential to foster or erode their sense of personal competence, uniqueness and, hence, personhood. This understanding promotes a shift from the disease process itself, to the interpersonal environment as the focus of change efforts. Countering the pessimism and hopelessness historically attached to working with 'the demented', the new vision offers exciting possibilities for positively influencing the dementia experience; neurological factors might not be readily modified but there is growing evidence that psychosocial interventions, environmental changes and assistive technologies can mitigate the extent of the disability and improve quality of life (see, for example, Kelly, 1993; Fratiglioni et al, 2000; Marshall, 2001; Bates et al, 2004; Fossey et al, 2006). While it is recognised that this evidence base is not without issues (Edvardsson et al, 2008), it nevertheless suggests that a focus on personhood offers hope and validates the importance of developing person-centred approaches to practice and research.

Second, this lens offers an important strategy for beginning to individualise the experience of dementia by contextualising it within a broader, lifecourse perspective. Kitwood (1992) perhaps articulated this most clearly, proposing that the clinical manifestation of dementia could be understood as arising from a complex interaction of five factors: personality (P), biography (B), physical health status (H), neurological impairment (NI) and social psychology (SP). He denoted this relationship using the equation: Dementia = P+B+H+NI+SP. Although Kitwood did not explicitly make the link between these factors and personhood, the underlying assumption is that they provide the foundation for addressing, promoting and respecting personhood. With this link, continuity between life experiences and the dementia experience is made that was previously missing. In particular, the importance of incorporating biographical knowledge about the person becomes critical for effectively understanding *each* person's unique experiences and fostering more effective, and humane, care. We need to know where people have come from and what they have lived through in order to understand who they are now (Bruce and Schweitzer, 2008).

Third, an approach that respects personhood has meant that the way people with dementia are spoken about and to has improved dramatically over the past 10 years. For example, until relatively recently, older people with dementia were often described as if they were living 'the death that leaves the body behind' or a 'social death' (Sweeting and Gilhooly, 1997), and therefore care providers were urged to 'look after the carer' since the person (with dementia) had, to all appearances, died and gone (Campbell et al, 1998). In addition, an individual with dementia was generally regarded as a 'sufferer' lacking insight into, and ability to articulate, their situation. This discourse silenced people with dementia: it provided no opportunities for people to speak. By drawing attention to personhood and the exclusion of the perspectives of people with dementia, the focus has shifted to incorporating the voices and understandings of people with dementia into both research and practice.

A result of this shift is that gradually research has begun to emerge aimed at capturing the perspectives of people with dementia (see, for example, Braudy-Harris, 2002a, 2002b; Wilkinson, 2002; Phinney, 2008). This body of research now clearly documents that people with dementia are often quite aware of their situation and can contribute important and unique insights about their experiences and needs (Bender and Cheston, 1997; Braudy-Harris, 2002b; Phinney and Chesla, 2003; Beard, 2004; Clare et al, 2005; Hirschman et al, 2005; Whitlatch et al, 2005). The net result is that since the introduction of personhood into the debate, research and practice has shifted from failing to even consider whether people with dementia have anything to say, to acknowledging that indeed they do, and recognising the importance of hearing their perspectives. Emphasis is now being placed on seeking creative and innovative strategies to overcome impaired communication associated with the condition in order to facilitate hearing these voices. Thus, the use of a personhood lens has effectively and explicitly brought the person with dementia into the picture.

For the above reasons, although there has been some critical debate about person-centred care, especially as conceptualised by Kitwood (see, for example, Adams, 1996; Parker, 2001; Nolan et al, 2002; Dewing, 2004, O'Connor et al, 2007), the notion of an intersubjective personhood is generally accepted as a useful lens for dementia practice and research.

Evidence of its impact is the significant changes over the past 10 years in health and social care policies, especially in the UK. For example, in the UK in the 1980s, people with dementia were implicitly positioned as a burden, a drain on health and social care resources (Health Advisory Service, 1983; Ineichen, 1987), and here, like elsewhere, supportive interventions concentrated almost entirely on the needs of caregivers (Cotrell and Schulz, 1993). More recently, however, UK health policy directives such as the National Dementia Strategy for England (DH, 2009), have explicitly recognised people with dementia as entitled to quality care and services. Consequently, there is a greater emphasis on user involvement in service planning and delivery, which has resulted in numerous studies that seek insights and feedback from people with dementia, as well as caregivers.

Recognising the boundaries of personhood

While attention to personhood in the dementia debate has achieved much in terms of raising consciousness about the intrinsic value of individuals with dementia and offering promise that constructive changes can be achieved, it has boundaries. Several issues emerge which are particularly relevant for positioning the need to broaden the vision. These will be organised around three core issues: how the person with dementia is positioned; how 'context' is actually contextualised; and (in)attention to power.

Positioning of the person with dementia

A significant boundary to how personhood has been utilised to date is that while it is grounded in the idea that a person with dementia is someone who counts, this lens does not necessarily promote the vision of someone with agency. Sociologists broadly define agency as the capacity of individuals to influence the circumstances in which they live (for a fuller discussion, see Emirbayer and Mische, 1998). It is an important concept as it emphasises the ability of individuals to reflect on and seek to change the social practices and forces they face. Human agency might be expressed cognitively – through language, for example – or it might be asserted in a more embodied way, through the control of feelings (Shilling, 1997) and use of bodily gestures (Kontos, 2005). Although arguably visible in Kitwood's earlier work (Baldwin and Capstick, 2007), noticeably missing in his discussion of personhood is any reference to agency. In *Dementia reconsidered*, for instance, Kitwood (1997a, pp 46/7) spoke about the way in which certain care practices (malignant social psychology) undermine personhood without any reference to the agency of people with dementia. The implicit assumption seemed to be that individuals are necessarily passive in the face of external forces.

Moreover, reinforcing a sense of passivity, personhood is conceptualised as something that is conferred on a person with dementia, conveying a uni-directional understanding that continues to position a person with dementia as dependent on others for affirmation. For example, Downs (1997, p 598) notes that maintaining the personhood of people with dementia essentially becomes 'the responsibility of those who are cognitively intact' rather than the individual with dementia. Dewing (2007) takes this a step further, commenting that personhood is seen as a status, rather than a continual process of recognition. Thus, a personhood lens does not explicitly recognise the status of a person with dementia as either intrinsic or self-enabled.

Another issue associated with how the person with dementia is positioned is that underpinning existing ways of understanding personhood is an implicit focus on *maintenance* of status, rather than growth, development and proliferation of statuses. Specifically, a core theme that dominates the person-centred literature highlights the importance of 'knowing' the person with dementia, including drawing on his/her biography and life experiences, to promote approaches that will maintain his/her personhood. This has been an important step forward. However, we have now reached somewhat of an impasse: how do we use this biographical material without allowing it to restrict opportunities for change? This issue can be especially well illustrated when we look at discussions around advanced care planning and directives where people with early dementia are increasingly encouraged to take control of their own care by planning for the future. In principle, this advice makes complete sense but new debates are now emerging regarding how valid advanced instructions actually are. Specifically, when talking in the abstract, many of us indicate that we would prefer death to life under certain conditions; however, when confronted with the actual situation at least some of these same people will cling tenaciously to life despite what was said from a position of health. The problem with dementia is that we do not know yet how to accommodate the notion that, like anyone else, people with dementia may change – they may change their mind, they may want to experiment, they may legitimately lose interest in activities that once enthralled them. The net result here is that to date, there has been a tendency to conceptualise personhood in a way that may inadvertently collude with the biomedical model to effectively discount people with dementia by relegating change to the neuropathological changes associated with the dementia rather than normal lifecourse maturation.

(De)contextualising the dementia experience

The shift from a cognitive-based understanding of personhood to one that is more relational has been a huge step forward. However, further boundaries emerge with the approach when the attempts to contextualise are critically examined. First, despite the rhetoric around an inter-subjective personhood, attention to personhood has retained an individualised lens for understanding the dementia experience. While the importance of the relationship for fostering, or impeding, personhood is highlighted, much of the literature still assumes a core individual concerned with autonomy and self-determination; 'person–centred care' and 'individualised care' are terms that are often used interchangeably. This is problematic at a number of levels, beginning with questions about the cultural appropriateness of the notion. As Tsai (2009) notes, an individualised perspective is less relevant in Eastern culture where familial relationships and community tend to be prioritised. Thus, personhood may be an important Western concept but its relevance beyond less individualistic societies has not been established.

The failure to adequately contextualise personhood has also led to concerns that a level of homogeneity in the dementia experience has been assumed that effectively mutes difference and limits the development of a textured understanding of the experiences (Downs, 2000; Hulko, 2002; Innes, 2002, 2009; Bond et al, 2004; O'Connor et al, 2007). Specifically, 'the dementia' is assumed to hold priority positioning over other aspects of social location such as age, gender, 'race', socioeconomic status and sexual orientation. How life with dementia is shaped and/or different depending on a person's social positions are questions that are only rarely asked. This is despite the fact that when they are asked, evidence is emerging which indicates that people's experiences of dementia vary depending on these other aspects. For example, Hulko (2009) found that people who could be classified as more privileged (based for example on socioeconomic status, gender and/or 'race') could be more devastated by the losses affiliated with the dementia than others who positioned it as 'no big deal' in the scheme of the bigger issues they contended with on a day-to-day basis. Others, for example Henderson and Traphagan (2005), describe how a person's cultural background offers diverse ways of making meaning of the dementia – they found that in some aboriginal communities the individual may be accorded heightened status within the community as someone who was in closer communication with the spirits. The tendency to talk about *the* dementia experience, rather than dementia experiences, is useful for bringing people together but it also has the unintended effect of failing to capture the complexities and tensions that construct all people's lives –

including those with dementia. In particular, it facilitates a sanitised understanding because it hides how other sources of disadvantage may impact the experiences.

This failure to adequately contextualise can also be seen in how 'social relationships' have been approached. Most frequently, emphasis has been limited to understanding experiences within the immediate interpersonal context. For example, a growing body of research has focused on articulating how people with dementia make sense of their diagnosis and cope with the cognitive changes (see Phinney, 2008 for a review of this body of research); this research has been instrumental in beginning to highlight individual coping strategies, responses and communication patterns. Simultaneously, considerable research has examined quality of care, with a particular emphasis on creating caring environments and relationships that are more respectful and responsive to the individual. The result has been that after 10 years of research involving people with dementia much is known about micro level issues such as quality of care, communication techniques and individual coping strategies, but less is known about macro level issues, including how to identify and eradicate discriminatory practices.

By restricting how 'social relationships' (Kitwood, 1997b) have been conceptualised to the interpersonal, a concern arises that responsibility for the treatment of people with dementia may simply have shifted from the disease process to the person's immediate environment. There are two issues here. First, this person now assumes power over the person with dementia. Second, blame can be assigned and there is no need to capture how wider social processes and systems influence what is, or is not, done. 'Agitated behaviour', for example, has now been attributed to poor treatment by care staff, instead of the 'diseased brain' explanation of the biomedical perspective, but organisational and societal practices and policies that may lead to poor treatment remain unexamined.

(In)attention to power

This previous point is not simply an issue of developing an incomplete picture related to inadequate contextualised understanding. Rather, it is linked to a third area where boundaries associated with personhood can most readily be identified: personhood has typically been framed apolitically. Personhood is an intuitively appealing term, concerned primarily with psychological and interpersonal relationships; as such, it does not readily provide the language for discussing people's situations in terms of power (as opposed to psychosocial) relations. In order to begin to change the culture of care, dementia care mapping (DCM) was developed, which measures the well-being and ill-being of the person with dementia, largely based on how the care staff interact with the person with dementia. While this is a valuable observation tool, it does not move from the focus on the interpersonal interaction to examine how a particular interaction is constructed by a broader institutional or societal focus. It fails to consider that these 'caring interactions' are initiated by care staff – usually female, often the most poorly paid, poorly educated and most marginalised group – within an organisational context often driven by for-profit, task-based priorities. In other words, how these interactions reflect power differentials is ignored. As Fox (1995) notes, a personhood lens does not have the language for exploring the possibility that 'caring' might sometimes have more to do with power and control than with values of trust and giving, nor is this lens really able to describe relationships in the context of wider social divisions. Baldwin and Capstick (2007) note that by treating dementia care organisations as though they are effectively 'hermeneutically sealed institutions separate from the rest of the social world and its economic agendas and priorities', the potential for change within the organisational level may be significantly overestimated (p 273). Consequently, sociopolitical matters such as experiences of discrimination – both by people with dementia and their carers – may be overlooked, and engagement in activities that have political (as well as personal) meaning are not seen or discussed as such.

The emergence of a fourth moment

The need to extend understanding of the dementia experience to capture a more dynamic, contextualised perspective is now emerging. Arguably, this represents an emerging fourth moment in dementia studies. Contained within this expanding vision are two critical and interrelated themes: the need for a bi-directional interactive understanding, that is, one that recognises that people with dementia are influenced by – but also influence (because they have agency) – interpersonal and social relationships; and the importance of a more textured, multidimensional lens for contextualising the experience, specifically one that incorporates the importance of sociocultural context. Developing a response to these two thematic imperatives provides the foundation for broadening the debate around dementia.

Of these two themes, the focus on a more interactive, dynamic approach has perhaps been best developed through discussions around 'relationship-centered care' (Nolan et al, 2006). This approach focuses on relational reciprocity, and has been described as having 'the potential to change the culture of dementia care in ways that ensure that the personhood of, and the interdependencies between, all stakeholders are protected and enhanced' (Davies and Nolan, 2008, p 438). It emphasises the importance of attending to the relationships between and among family members, people with dementia and formal caregivers as an essential element of quality dementia care. The model makes explicit the importance of interconnectedness and partnerships. Given this, it represents an important extension in the personhood focus because it captures expectations that the person with dementia will retain status as an active partner in the dementia experience. It begins to move beyond a uni-directional account into one that is more dynamic and interactive.

However, while this approach has indeed broadened the debate, there is still distance to cover. Specifically, with few exceptions, the focus remains on care relationships as opposed to the other relationships people have, such as those with the state and its institutions; this means that implicitly the person with dementia continues to be positioned largely as one who needs care (despite the recognition that there is some interdependency within the caring relationship). Moreover, although the person with dementia is recognised as having expertise over his/her own body and experiences, the thrust of this approach has tended to be on professional support to facilitate positive relationships. In other words, although fundamentally congruent to a dynamic approach, it is unclear how the expertise and agency of the person with dementia is actually being considered. Finally, the need to grapple with how relationships and experiences are grounded by broader sociocultural context remains unaddressed.

Attempts to develop this more contextualised understanding are now emerging. O'Connor and colleagues at the Centre for Research on Personhood in Dementia (CRPD) (O'Connor et al, 2007) suggest one framework. They propose a three-dimensional model that positions personhood at the nexus of subjective experience (SE), interactional environment (IE) and sociocultural context (SCC). In this model:

- subjective experience refers to the perceptions and meanings of the person with dementia;
- interactional environment is used to capture the focus on the importance of a person's interactions with others but extends it to recognise that personal relationships are only one aspect of the immediate environment within which the person with dementia interacts on a day-to-day basis. Other aspects such as the use of physical space and engagement in activities also provide interactional opportunities which can either foster or erode a person's sense of personal competence and uniqueness, and hence personhood; and
- sociocultural context recognises the different levels of contextual embedding that shape dementia experiences. These include, for example: organisational or systemic policies and practices, social location (which reflects a person's position within sociocultural groupings and includes, but is not limited to ethnic positioning, gender, socioeconomic positioning) and broader societal discourses such as those that help shape our understanding of the importance of autonomy, independence and cognitive functioning.

The advantage of this framework is that it makes explicit the importance of broadening the 'relational' component beyond interpersonal relationships to consider how these are shaped and constructed within a broader societal context. We note that this is not inconsistent with relationship-centred care; rather it is an extension that visibly ensures consideration of broader contexts. As noted by Innes (2009), this model assists in conceptualising research and practice at the micro level (subjective experience), mezzo level (interactional environment) and macro level (sociocultural context).

Drawing on the work of O'Connor et al (2009) and discussions with other CRPD researchers, Figure 2.1 adapts and develops this model still further to propose a more embedded, interactive framework.

Figure 2.1: A multidimensional model for contextualising dementia

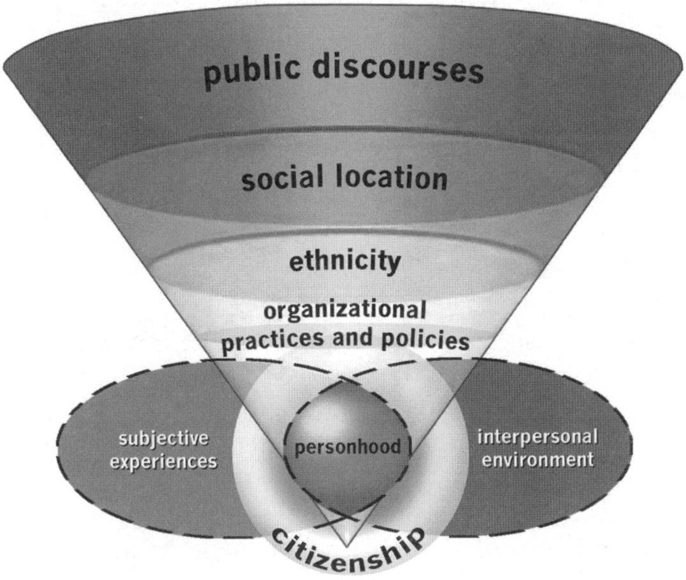

public discourses

social location

ethnicity

organizational
practices and policies

subjective
experiences

personhood

interpersonal
environment

citizenship

Source: Adapted from O'Connor et al (2007)

This adapted model develops the original model proposed by O'Connor et al (2007) in three ways. First, while it draws on the same multidimensional construction as the original, it graphically repositions the dimensions in order to recognise how embedded personal experiences and interpersonal relationships are within a broader societal context.

Second, it explicitly recognises the multiple layering associated with sociocultural contextualising. Specifically, the emerging framework tries to capture the complexity associated with conceptualising what is meant by 'sociocultural context' by recognising the various levels of abstraction that can be associated with the notion of culture (O'Connor et al, 2009). For example, a simplistic understanding of culture equates it with ethnicity or 'race'. However, when the notion of cultural contextualising is discursively broadened, the importance of understanding the systems of beliefs, assumptions and values that are being drawn on offers a potentially more useful, and expansive, understanding of cultural contextualising. This way of conceptualising sociocultural context begins to offer a lens both for understanding how 'subjective experience' is shaped by a person's social location, what ideas people draw on to construct their relationships with others, but also for analysing how particular values, beliefs and assumptions are enacted at broader organisational, systemic and societal levels. Re-configuring culture is important as it offers different places and ways for intervening and making change.

Third, this adaptation draws attention to the dynamic, multidirectional nature of the relationships among the three dimensions. This is critical to a social citizenship lens because it makes explicit that people with dementia *do* have power and *do* influence their interpersonal and social relationships.

This model, then, offers a framework for centring social citizenship as a critical concept in the dementia debate. In this fourth moment of dementia studies – one where sociopolitical context becomes more visible – social citizenship emerges as an exciting and important concept for expanding thinking and practice.

Conclusion

In the past 30 years dementia studies have undergone tremendous growth and development. Dementia has moved from being understood primarily (solely?) as a biomedical issue, to recognising the importance of understanding how a person's treatment within their personal and social relationships may impact functioning and retention of a sense of self.

Personhood has emerged as a core concept within this approach and much of the emphasis of this body of literature has been on the immediate interpersonal environment; considerably less attention has focused on embedding responses and relationships within a broader societal context. It is now time to extend the dialogue to begin to redress this imbalance. This chapter proposes a framework, based on the work of O'Connor et al (2007) at the CRPD for beginning to conceptualise this shift in thinking in a way that potentially captures a more sociopolitical perspective. This framework helps to position the importance of social citizenship as an essential concept that is beginning to emerge in dementia studies as a necessary adjunct to personhood. An analysis of a social citizenship lens is developed in Chapter Three.

THREE

The meaning and value of social citizenship

Introduction

In the previous chapter the argument was made for a more contextualised, sociopolitical understanding of dementia. In taking this approach, citizenship emerges as an essential concept. The concept of citizenship is proving increasingly popular among people with early dementia, service providers, professional care workers, voluntary organisations and academics alike, and is often used alongside personhood to promote the rights of people with dementia. However, it is generally used uncritically and with little explanation or clarification as to what it actually means in relation to people with dementia, especially individuals with very severe dementia. The aim of this chapter is to analyse the concept of citizenship, explore some of its strengths and boundaries and in so doing posit a way of understanding and defining social citizenship that has relevance for dementia studies.

The chapter begins by outlining a traditional view of citizenship before discussing contemporary definitions and analysis of this concept. The discussion focuses on contemporary definitions most relevant to people with dementia, including: citizenship as practice; active and passive modes of citizenship; the importance of recognising difference, contradiction and fragmentation; and semi-citizenship. Some of the boundaries of citizenship are outlined. In addition, the idea is compared and contrasted with personhood in order to show the elements that citizenship brings to the field. Having examined a range of debates about citizenship, and discussed it in relation to personhood, the chapter sets out the components of a social citizenship approach for dementia studies and concludes by arguing for further debate about the exact nature of citizenship in the context of people with dementia.

Traditional views of citizenship

The original idea of citizenship can be traced back to Aristotle, the Roman Empire and developments of the state. At that time the term was used to distinguish between those who were 'good citizens' and those who were not. Essentially, a 'good citizen' was considered to be someone who was politically active, full of civic spirit and educated, whereas a 'bad citizen' was someone who showed no interest in civic life or the workings of the state (Heater, 1999).

Modern views of citizenship can be dated back to the French Revolution in the mid–18th century when the idea was linked with equality and inalienable rights (Turner, 1986). At this point the use of citizenship changed; as Heater (2004, p 251) explains, it 'mutated from being an agent of segregation to one of association', so rather than using citizenship to 'differentiate between inhabitants' it became a means of 'equalising their status'.

Although the use of citizenship may have changed over time, it has fundamentally always been about the relationships individuals have with the state over the course of their life. Every citizen is linked to the state in one way or another, for example, as a taxpayer, voter, benefit claimant, consumer of public services and so forth. These links lie at the heart of a traditional view of citizenship and yet they are rarely explicitly discussed in dementia studies: the focus has been on familial relations or people's relationships with professional care workers as opposed to their identities vis-à-vis the state. Recognising the state as an inextricable domain of citizenship, or to put it another way, seeing government decisions and policies as a key influence in a person's life, is important because it highlights how lived experience and opportunities will inevitably be shaped by the rules, laws and policies of the country or jurisdiction in which a person lives. The following, well-publicised case of British couple Barbara and Malcolm Pointon illustrates how the state, and its various mechanisms influences people's lives:

> Malcolm Pointon was diagnosed with Alzheimer's disease in 1991. Seven years later he and his wife Barbara were offered a fully-funded NHS place in a care home. However, the home was too dark and Malcolm, because of his visuo-spatial difficulties, kept bumping into things. His wife found a more suitable care home for him but as the then health authority would not allow the NHS funding to follow him she had to personally fund the large gap between means-tested benefits and what the care actually cost. In 2001, Barbara Pointon lodged a formal complaint with her local Primary Care Trust, which eventually reached the Health Ombudsman. She complained that neither she nor her husband were receiving the services they were entitled to under the 1977 National Health Service Act; 1990 National Health Service and Community Care Act; and the 2000 Carers and Disabled Children's Act. The Pointons won their case and in 2003 the Primary Care Trust took over the full costs of Malcolm's care. He died at home in February, 2007. (Pointon, 2007)

The Pointon's case shows not only how the state influences our lives, but also how its mechanisms (that is, legislation) can be brought to bear in order to secure rights as a citizen.

One of the most well-known traditional views of citizenship was formulated by T.H. Marshall in the context of postwar Britain. At that time citizenship became defined as a 'status bestowed on those who are full members of a community.

All who possess the status are equal with respect to the rights and duties which the status bestows' (Marshall, 1949/92, p 18). A citizen was thus defined by the acquisition of, and participation in or membership of, the country or community in which they lived (Gould, 1988). With this view, citizenship involves three strands: civil, political and social rights and responsibilities. Briefly, the civil strand entails 'liberty of the person' and 'right to own property'; the political denotes the right to participate in democratic processes; and the social recognises the 'right to live the life of a civilised being' (Marshall and Hunter, 1992, quoted in Heater, 1999, p 13). This definition has evoked widespread criticism (some of which will be discussed later in this chapter); nevertheless, it remains one of the most influential views of citizenship today. One possible reason for its enduring appeal is because of its emphasis on social inequality and attempt to address this through the formulation of social rights in respect to issues including welfare (Dwyer, 2004).

Some boundaries of a traditional view of citizenship

A traditional view of citizenship is not without boundaries or drawbacks. One criticism levelled at Marshall's formulation is that it overlooks the existence and influences of social movements and citizen-inspired struggles. The emphasis is on how the state and its systems and institutions maintain and promote citizenship, rather than on how individuals and groups might do so through threats or acts of protests and hostility (Turner, 1990). This is unfortunate, as it means key moments in a group's claim for social citizenship are overlooked; think, for example, how British people with dementia took part in public demonstrations over the proposed withdrawal of anti-dementia drugs (BBC, 2007), while many others took part in a letter-writing campaign to Members of Parliament (MPs) on the same issue (SDWG, 2007). A very traditional view of citizenship fails to take account of citizen-driven campaigns for social change and is thus somewhat limited when it comes to understanding citizenship in the 21st century.

A second major drawback from a dementia studies perspective is the 'exclusionary tendency' of traditional views of citizenship (Lister, 2007, p 50). The way citizenship is commonly perceived, as a status with associated rights but also responsibilities, has a tendency to exclude those who for whatever reason are unable to claim their rights or fulfil their obligations as citizens. For example, a Marshallian view of citizenship presumes that every citizen is fully cognisant with the capacity to make judgements and decisions, assume responsibility, participate in the exercise of political power and fulfil civic obligations such as voting and working. The possibility that some citizens will not be cognitively able to do this, such as those with severe dementia, is rarely acknowledged or considered. Moreover, if it is thought about, this view of citizenship would disregard such people as non-citizens. This shows how essentialist or absolutist traditional views of citizenship can be: to be a citizen you must be cognitively able, there is no grey area in between, nor any context in which cognition is not deemed to be necessary.

These implicit assumptions underpinning a traditional view of citizenship make it virtually unworkable for dementia studies.

A third drawback of a traditional view of citizenship, related to its 'exclusionary tendency', is that it overlooks difference. It denies difference, not only in terms of the characteristics of being a citizen but also in terms of the rights and responsibilities that a citizen might expect and want. For example, some people will feel strongly about the right to be told if they have a dementia diagnosis, others will not. Similarly, some people will want to exercise their right to vote in local and general elections for as long as possible into the illness, but others will not see this as important at all. As one feminist notes, in a traditional view of citizenship it is assumed that every citizen wants and should be obligated to have and do the same thing, 'rights are represented as essentially abstract and universal and therefore not very amenable to a politics of difference' (Lister, 2003, p 87). Clearly, the field does not need an approach to citizenship that denies difference.

The problem with overlooking difference is that it denies the variations that exist between not only individual citizens, but also between and within countries. In the UK, for instance, currently only those living in Wales are entitled to free prescriptions; residents of England, Northern Ireland and Scotland have to meet certain eligibility criteria for this entitlement. In the US, people's rights and responsibilities in respect of healthcare would be very different again. Ignoring difference is a serious shortcoming of a traditional view of citizenship.

Citizenship as a social practice

In recent years, theorists have sought to address some of the boundaries of citizenship by changing the conceptual focus from legal rights and civic responsibilities to the social practice of citizenship (see, for example, Shotter, 1993; Barnes, 1997; Barnes et al 2004; Isin and Wood, 1999; Lister, 2003).

This change in focus redefines citizenship as not only a status which has an attached series of actual or assumed rights, but also as a social practice through which individuals relate to other people, their communities and the state (Prior et al, 1995). Table 3.1 outlines some of the ways in which citizenship is defined as a social practice.

With this perspective, the notion of citizenship is more broadly defined so, rather than it being a status bestowed 'from above', namely the state, citizenship is achieved by individuals or groups in a social context through the power dynamics of everyday talk and actions (Barnes et al, 2004). Citizenly practices thus become more dyadic and readily found in everyday life. For instance, a woman with dementia who seems to lack purpose when at home with her husband, but who is active and tremendously helpful and supportive to both staff and other clients at the adult day centre (Sabat, 2003, p 7), can be seen as a form of social citizenship.

Although such actions are more commonly viewed through a personhood lens, the key to recognising social citizenship as a practice is to consider what a person does and with what *public* consequences (Lister, 2007, p 57; emphasis added).

Table 3.1: Competing definitions of citizenship as a practice

Definition	Source
Satisfying demands for full inclusion into social community	Pakulski (1997)
'Citizenship as the expression of human agency'	Lister (2003, p 39)
'Citizenship is a set of norms, values and practices designed to solve collective action problems'	Pattie, Seyd and Whitely (2004, p 22)
Acts of citizenship are fundamental ways of being with others	Isin and Nielsen (2008)
'Citizenship is one of the primary ways in which individuals 'realize' (in both senses of the word) their identities as civic and political agents'	Barnes, Auburn and Lea (2004, p189)
'Citizenship offers the opportunity to participate in one's own life and in the creation and re-creation of the conditions within which that life is acted out'	(Clarke, 1996, p 26)

In this case, for example, the public consequence was an additional (voluntary) pair of hands for the day care centre and a role model to which other users of the centre might aspire. Other acts of social citizenship, such as the campaign by Barbara Pointon on behalf of her husband Malcolm, can have more far-reaching consequences – in this case, the primary care trust reviewed its continuing care criteria, and Barbara's campaign sparked a public debate in the UK about the rights of people with dementia to fully funded healthcare. Thinking about citizenship as a social practice is helpful as it broadens how the actions of people with dementia might be interpreted, and it opens up dialogue about the wider consequences of people's actions.

Recognising difference, contradiction and fragmentation

The trend towards a social practice of citizenship reflects postmodernist ideas for understanding citizenship. Postmodernism defies definition as it is a way of understanding the social world that contests structure, categories and meaning (Bauman, 1992). For example, the mini-mental state examination (MMSE) would be perceived as too standardised and simplistic a tool using a more postmodernistic lens. A postmodernist lens recognises difference, contradiction and fragmentation – different, contradictory and fragmented identities, beliefs, values, sexualities, lifestyles, cultures, worldviews, meanings, narratives – indeed, any issue related to the human experience (Bartlett and O'Connor, 2007). This take on citizenship is exciting, as it recognises the messiness of human life, as well as the challenges of trying to understand people's struggles and experiences of citizenship. Unlike the traditional view of citizenship, with its lofty assumptions and ideals about what it means to be a citizen, this way of thinking about citizenship recognises that there is no fixed or proper way of being a citizen. Instead, people are seen as having multiple identities and social roles, making up their citizenly status (Faulks, 2000).

Recognising difference, contradiction and fragmentation is an important conceptual shift, particularly for dementia studies, as a person's status as a citizen is forged in part through 'struggles around differentiated identities' and membership to social groups (Lister, 2003, p 15). With this perspective, there is no right or wrong way of being a citizen, or of being 'a person with dementia', as individuals and groups are shaping and determining their own status and citizen identity. Some of the contradictions inherent in this process are coming to light in the field. For example, Beard (2004) discusses how organisations like the Alzheimer's Association have to portray dementia in a very negative, medical way (in order to 'garner public sympathy') while at the same time support those with dementia who are advocating for themselves to achieve a different picture. This is what one of Beard's respondents said:

> What we have to do is make sure we're protecting human rights at the same time we're letting the world know how awful and ugly and destructive the disease is. Separating the human, the person, from the disease is a trick because you need the person to exhibit the disease. (public policy spokesperson, quoted in Beard, 2004, p 806)

(Re)determining the status and identities of people with dementia is clearly a complex and inherently contradictory process. This becomes critical to recognise if we are to avoid the trap of essentialising some aspects of a person, and 'boxing them' into categories that are limiting.

Active and passive modes of citizenship

Another important conceptual advance in debates about citizenship that is particularly relevant to dementia studies is the idea of active and passive modes of citizenship. Initially it was Ignatieff (1989) who advanced this distinction, defining active modes in terms of running for political office, voting and so forth, and passive modes in terms of entitlement to rights and welfare. In traditional accounts of citizenship non-action tends to be seen in a pejorative way: as a sign of a second-class or 'non'-citizen. However, distinguishing between an active and passive mode means that it is not degree of participation that defines someone as a citizen of the state. Rather it is the degree to which a person's rights are recognised and upheld. The best way to show this is to explain in more detail and consider some examples of active and passive modes.

Active participation is most often associated with the overtly political, that is, taking part in some form of democratic process such as voting, political forums and/or the development of public policies. The involvement of people with dementia in the National Dementia Strategy for England (DH, 2009) is an example of this kind of political participation. People with dementia helped design the strategy and are now a part of the Reference Group set up to ensure it is implemented. Other forms of active citizenship are less public and connected to state processes but are nevertheless still concerned with making a difference. For example, an older resident in a care home who takes a role in the management, day-to-day running and social life of that home through, for example, participation on the resident's council, is engaging in an active form of citizenship.

Active citizenship, then, is not simply about a person getting involved in everyday life; it is about that person making and participating in decisions that affect not only their own life, but also the lives of those around them. We have outlined some of the more collective and formal ways in which people do this, but individuals with dementia are also making decisions and being active citizens in many other ways; for example: taking part in fundraising events for charities like the Alzheimer's Society; making donations; writing letter to MPs; making consumer choices about which service to use; and lodging a formal complaint, or indeed compliment, about the quality of care. All these activities are important not only to the person with dementia, but also society at large. On this count, the notion of active citizenship offers a piece that has been occurring, but not necessarily discussed, in the field of dementia studies.

In contrast, passive modes of citizenship are concerned with people getting what they are entitled to or have a right to expect as an equal citizen. For example, a person with very severe dementia who is dying is entitled to pain relief and other palliative care measures; receipt of these would be to experience a passive mode of citizenship, and would not constitute a loss of citizenship. Similarly, in Britain, certain citizens, including those over the age of 60, and those registered as severely sight impaired/blind or sight impaired/partially sighted, are entitled to a free sight test under the NHS. If a person is denied access to an optician because they have a dementia diagnosis, say, or they live in a care home, this would constitute a passive infringement of their citizenship.

The notion of passive citizenship is consistent in some ways with how personhood has been used and adapted within the dementia literature. It seeks to ensure a person receives the treatment and support they are entitled to in a timely, dignified and respectful manner. The link between personhood and citizenship will be further discussed later in this chapter. However, two important differences will be highlighted here.

First, citizenship is rights-based, not needs-based. This means that if a person is denied a treatment or service on the basis of a social category – such as age, dementia diagnosis or ethnicity – that person will have clearer, more concrete, grounds on which to complain. This is less explicit when discussing personhood. Second, passive citizenship clearly provides a language that takes into account how social inequalities, such as age, gender, disability, ethnicity, social class, sexuality, neighbourhood, marital status and so forth may form the foundation for discrimination. Again, this is not so clear when thinking about personhood.

One inequality we know impacts on the passive citizenship of people with dementia relates to the stigma attached to the label 'Alzheimer's disease' or 'dementia'. Valuable work has been done in this area but it is usually from an individual's perspective and not necessarily debated in the context of passive citizenship (see, for example, Alzheimer's Society, 2008). Thinking about stigma through the lens of passive citizenship you can see how it is a structural issue. Take, for example, the inequities surrounding the use of prescription drugs. Cholinesterase inhibitors (such as donepezil and galantamine), which are known to help people with dementia, can only be prescribed freely under the NHS (in England, Wales and Northern Ireland) to those in the moderate stages of Alzheimer's disease. People without a diagnosis of Alzheimer's disease, or those in the very early or late stages of the illness, are not entitled to these drugs at all. Conversely, drugs which have potentially harmful effects, namely, antipsychotics, are given to a 'worryingly' high number of people with dementia – up to a quarter of people with dementia in the UK are prescribed these drugs, the majority of whom will be in a care home (Banerjee, 2009, p 20). The idea of passive citizenship draws attention to the unjust and discriminatory nature of prescribing practices like these. Consistent with the notion of citizenship in general, the focus is on the *grounds* on which people are denied and/or afforded services and treatments, and not just whether or not they are seen as a person. Moreover, passive citizenship, realises that not all citizens will be in a position that they are able to actively assert these rights.

Thinking in terms of passive and active modes means citizenship becomes as much about 'recognition as about access to formal rights' (Lister, 2007, p 51), recognition of not only the personhood of all human beings but also their particular circumstances and social situation. Critically, it means that those who may lack the cognisance or physical ability to actively participate in civic life are not disenfranchised; even if someone is unable to participate as a citizen in a conventionally active or political way, they are still seen and treated as a citizen.

Notion of semi-citizenship

Another way that the concept of citizenship is being adapted so that it is potentially more inclusive of people with dementia is through the notion of semi-citizenship. Cohen (2009) introduced the notion of semi-citizenship in an attempt to clarify the ways in which certain social groups, such as people with disabilities, are citizens by some standards and not others. As the term denotes, it paves the way for a middle ground between being a full citizen and non-citizen, and encourages the unpacking of citizenship as a concept in order to see which elements of citizenship are important for which groups. This conceptualisation of social citizenship is perhaps the first to address the paradox that some individuals in society are simply not able to uphold the full status of democratic citizenship (for example, babies, young children and the very severely impaired), but they are citizens nevertheless. The field of dementia studies should keep abreast of how this conceptualisation of social citizenship develops.

Social citizenship and people with dementia

Citizenship is a strategic and evolving concept. New conceptualisations have ensured that the concept has particular currency for dementia studies. Growing recognition of its relevance is apparent in the myriad of ways that different individuals and groups have used it to denote and promote various aspects of living with dementia. For example, members of the Scottish Dementia Working Group (SDWG) use it to campaign for better services and treatment; Lynda Hogg said, "citizenship for me means being a full member of society, being treated equally and having choices" (quoted in SDWG, 2007); academics have used it to strengthen the idea that people have rights especially in regard to decisions about their care (see, for example, Boyle, 2008); and service providers have drawn on the notion to re-emphasise a person's innate right to belong (Judd, 2007). In most instances citizenship is being used to reawaken interest in people with dementia, with a goal to make visible the potential injustices that this group face.

However, as stated at the start of this chapter, whenever citizenship is used in the dementia debate, its meaning is often taken for granted or only explained in the particular context of care. One possible reason for this is because the utility of this concept for transforming practice has yet to be fully conceptualised or explained.

A working definition of social citizenship for dementia studies

Given the different ways of defining and conceptualising citizenship, and the current lack of clarity in the field around this concept, we will begin by proposing a working definition of citizenship to use in relation to people with dementia. The rationale for providing a working definition is not to simplify a very complex issue, but rather to at least provide a common foundation from which to jump off by making it clear what we consider are the key components of social citizenship. This helps open the concept up to closer scrutiny and provides direction on how to locate it. The following is offered as a working definition:

Social citizenship can be defined as a relationship, practice or status, in which a person with dementia is entitled to experience freedom from discrimination, and to have opportunities to grow and participate in life to the fullest extent possible. It involves justice, recognition of social positions and the upholding of personhood, rights and a fluid degree of responsibility for shaping events at a personal and societal level.

Unlike a traditional view of citizenship the critical issue with this understanding is not just with rights and responsibilities but whether people with dementia have a potential and equal stake in all aspects of private and public life.

Contrast with personhood

In order to highlight its definitional qualities still further, a traditional view of citizenship can be compared and contrasted with personhood. The idea of having a 'status bestowed' is not new to dementia studies, and indeed resembles Kitwood's definition of personhood (Bartlett and O'Connor, 2007). Thus, the two concepts have a similar epistemological base. However, a fundamental difference between personhood and citizenship is that discussions about citizenship are by implication discussions about power, and in particular, the lack of power afforded to some citizens in relation to others. In this sense, as already noted, citizenship has deeper implications than personhood because it moves into the realm of political discourse – particularly the idea that participation or inclusion in society is inevitably shaped by power dynamics (Thomas, 2004). Table 3.2 outlines the contrasting elements of personhood, traditional and postmodern citizenship and illustrates how each lens promotes a different understanding of human experience. Personhood and citizenship have different historical roots, so it is not surprising that the two have distinctly different emphasis from one another (Bartlett and O'Connor, 2007). For example, from a legal/philosophical perspective a personhood lens has typically resulted in questions regarding whether or not people with dementia can have personhood (see for example, Davis, 2004) whereas a discussion of citizenship assumes personhood but queries the set of rights and responsibilities affiliated with that status. Each also brings a different perspective on experience. Personhood emphasises the uniqueness of human experience whereas citizenship is traditionally associated with the idea of a collective experience, and championing what people share – or should share – most notably, an 'equality of status' and opportunities (Marshall, 1949/92, cited in Dwyer, 2004, p 40).

The point of contrasting citizenship with personhood in this way is not to polarise debate within the field of dementia studies, or to imply that citizenship is somehow a superior concept to personhood. On the contrary, as demonstrated in Figure 2.1 in Chapter Two, personhood and citizenship are intertwined and are

Table 3.2: Contrasting elements of personhood, modern and postmodern citizenship

	Personhood	Modern citizenship	Postmodern citizenship
Historical roots	Psychology, moral philosophy	Political philosophy	Cultural politics
Emphasis	Needs-based	Rights and responsibilities	Practices
Position of self	Singular	Collective	Multifaceted/ multidimensional
Conferment of status	Moral, ethical	Constitutional	Social/semi
Type of experience	Unique (individual)	Common (shared)	Contextual

Source: Adapted from Bartlett and O'Connor (2007)

both important to the field and to understanding dementia. However, by teasing out the differences between these two concepts it is possible to show what each one brings to debate, and most critically, to highlight the potential of citizenship, as a sociopolitical concept, for broadening dementia debate.

Towards a conceptual framework of social citizenship in dementia

At several points in this book the need to go beyond care and psychological issues has been emphasised and the importance of reconsidering the situation of people with dementia from a wider sociopolitical perspective has been raised. In this section a broader conceptual framework for dementia studies is developed: the aim is to facilitate and stimulate the expansion of such thinking and practice.

A conceptual framework is a structured collection of ideas for understanding a given phenomenon; such frameworks often simultaneously act as a stimulus for debate. The framework presented in this section integrates key ideas from both dementia and citizenship studies, and seeks to understand and stimulate debate about the entitlements and actions of citizens with dementia in the broadest sense. The focus is on the actual components of the framework – what it looks like, and in particular, how it synthesises key ideas and extends current debates in the dementia field. The practical application of this framework will be outlined in Part II.

The conceptual framework proposed is a simple one consisting of six components: growth, social positions, purpose, participation, community and freedom from discrimination. The starting point for each of these components is a key idea from Kitwood's approach to dementia care, namely, a person's need for comfort, identity, occupation, inclusion, attachment and love, as outlined and depicted in the shape of a flower (Kitwood, 1997a, p 82). Some of these ideas have already evolved through the development of the SENSES framework that shifts from a person-centred approach to one that is more relationally grounded. The SENSES framework is built around the importance of a sense of: security, continuity, belonging, purpose, achievement and significance (Ryan et al, 2008). We build further onto this work, particularly Kitwood's framework, by extending thinking towards a conceptual framework of social citizenship that recognises the person with dementia as an active agent with rights, history and competencies. Figure 3.1 depicts this shift.

From comfort to growth

Feeling comfortable in both body and mind, and experiencing human tenderness and warmth are central to well-being (Kitwood, 1997a). This is indisputable: our need for comfort is primal. Further, it is important that people with dementia experience a sense of security in terms of feeling physically fine and free from harm or threat (Ryan et al, 2008). This too is vital, particularly in the context of

Figure 3.1: Extending the continuum of concepts for understanding people's actions and experiences

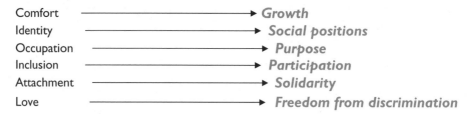

The point is, when talking about the well-being of people with dementia, it does not make sense to restrict the focus to comfort and a sense of psychological security; it places boundaries on, and narrows our understanding of the situation and practices of people with dementia. Moreover, it leaves the field without a structure or language for theorising the ways in which people with dementia seek to develop, experiment and grow as citizens.

a caring relationship. However, if a social citizenship approach is taken, comfort and a sense of security are not enough in and of themselves to strive for; people must also have opportunities to grow.

Opportunities for growth may take many forms. For example, they could be political in nature, and involve developing into an effective advocate, as is the case with people like Jim Mann, Richard Taylor and Lynn Jackson. Or they might be more artistic or spiritual in nature, as is the case with artist Rex Marsden:

> Following a diagnosis of vascular dementia, Rex Marsden began to lose 'his assertive business character and became more relaxed and in harmony with his situation. Despite a tremor in his right hand (due to Parkinson's) his painting improved immensely as each day was focused on two or three hours painting'. (quote taken directly from Rex Marsden's website, www.rexmarsden.co.uk)

The point is, when talking about the well-being of people with dementia, it does not make sense to restrict the focus to comfort and a sense of psychological security; it places boundaries on, and narrows our understanding of the situation and practices of people with dementia. Moreover, it leaves the field without a structure or language for theorising the ways in which people with dementia seek to develop, experiment and grow as citizens.

Feeling comfortable and secure in both body and mind is not only about the avoidance of pain and distress, but also about having opportunities to grow as human beings. In the context of social citizenship the idea of 'growth' is an important one, as it recognises a person's inner hopes, desires and capacity to contribute to life. From this perspective 'growth' means to be able to develop different aspects of oneself in the context of having one aspect deteriorating. For example, some couples report how their relationship has grown as a result of one partner having dementia (Braudy-Harris, 2002b, p 12). Similarly, one small group of men and women with dementia were clearly energised and able to develop creative skills when they became involved in a photography project (Mitchell, 2005). Introducing the idea of growth into the dementia debate broadens the spectrum of experiences and actions that can be explored. It also moves us another step away from the discourse of loss and despair that can be so overwhelming when talking about dementia.

From identity to social positions

There has been much debate about identity in relation to people with dementia (see, for example, work by Harris and Sterin, 1999; Sabat, 2001; and Surr, 2006). Early debates focused on whether or not a person with dementia was able to retain a sense of identity or 'self'. Initially it was (wrongly) assumed that the onset of dementia inevitably led to the complete loss of self. This view has now been successfully challenged and is no longer accepted. Instead, more current views recognise that a person's identity is unique and co-constructed (Kitwood, 1997a, p 84), and thus loss of identity is a potential hazard, rather than an inevitable consequence, of the condition (Bruce and Schweitzer, 2008).

The debate has recently shifted again from concerns about *whether* people retain a sense of self to *how* identity is maintained (see, for example, Clare et al, 2008). This is reflected in the SENSES framework by recognising and promoting the importance of a sense of continuity for older people, including those with dementia (Ryan et al, 2008). However, there are underlying epistemological problems associated with discussions about 'identity' that are relevant to conceptualising social citizenship. Some of these have already been recognised in the existing dementia literature and are now outlined.

First, at its most fundamental level, the notion of 'an identity' is problematic because it implicitly rests on essentialist understandings of a fixed, or owned, sense of 'self': a person has 'an identity', or a set of characteristics, which essentially remains unchanged, regardless of context or wider politics. This introduces questions about the possibility of change. More than this, however, it fails to acknowledge the multiple identities, or positions that a person with dementia may occupy. Others have recognised this concern. For example, Lyman (1998) has argued how dementia is just one aspect of a person's identity, not their only or primary identity. A person with dementia – like all people – holds identities that are shaped by their age, ethnicity, familial positions (such as aunt, grandfather), sexuality and so forth. Sabat's work (2001; see also Sabat and Harre, 1992) has been especially useful for helping to move beyond a static understanding of identity to one that is more fluid and layered, as has the work by high profile people with dementia (see, for example, presentations by DASNI [Dementia Advocacy and Support Network International] members at www.dasninternational.org/).

Certainly work on the diversity of people's lives points to the need to move beyond a singular identity to recognise multiple identities. However, simply pluralising this component is not sufficient. The second shortcoming with the identity (identities, even) related debate is that too frequently it leads to discussions about a person's 'role' that do not in any way address power relations. Take, for example, the situation of someone with dementia whom we will call Mrs Long. Mrs Long is recognised as a retired schoolteacher who enjoyed playing golf and bridge. This picture helps the observer 'know' Mrs Long but it does little to reposition her as someone with rights. Here the notion of 'status' extends discussions about identities. It is important to recognise who Mrs Long is, but it is also important to recognise the status – or lack of status – that is associated with various identities, or positions, that she holds. In our present society, one aspect of a person's identity, that of a person with dementia, routinely results in the downgrading of a person's status as an equal citizen.

Thinking in terms of multiple identities is advantageous as it reinforces the idea that there are many ways for a person with dementia to be in the social world. Moving beyond it to talk about status opens up discourse about lifecourse, and in particular, the impact of social structures – like age – on 'processes of identification' (Hockey and James, 2003, p 20). However, there is still a third shortcoming related to current understandings around identity. Specifically, when a person's identities are formed in relation to their different positions within the world, unsurprisingly there will be points of tension. Different positions hold different status and these will work in tandem with and opposition to one another: a middle-aged white male with dementia may have elevated status in comparison with an immigrant older woman.

The point here is to recognise that discussions about identity, while important, are conceptually inadequate. New language and ways of thinking are required to capture the complexities of people's social location in the world, and how these are reflected in terms of rights and responses. As one start to this process we are suggesting that the notion of 'social positions' is conceptually richer and more useful to a social citizenship framework than the notion of an identity.

From occupation to purpose

A person's need for occupation is well established in not only the dementia field but in health sciences generally. Much has been written about the benefits of occupying people with dementia with meaningful activities, such as cooking, preparing meals, reminiscing. Further, the importance of finding out about a person's previous occupation in order to individualise such activities is widely recognised as good practice. However, in the dementia debate, 'occupation' is usually quite narrowly defined and discussed only in terms of its psychosocial or therapeutic value. Moreover, the tendency in the field has often been to create and speak of 'artificial' environments such as 'cookery' classes, or 'therapy' sessions related to activities such as dance, art, reminiscing and music rather than to see such activities through a broader everyday lens. Think, for example, about how outings for care home residents are often conceptualised as 'meeting care needs' rather than as providing opportunities for people to access facilities in their local community that they are entitled to use – for example, museums, libraries, parks, adult education courses. The same can be said of conceptualisations about occupation within the SENSES framework, where a sense of purpose is still very much linked with therapeutic goals.

A further limitation of the term 'occupation' is that it is closely aligned to the notion of 'doing' rather than meaning and so there is no space to debate the different values and ways of being in the world that a person with dementia might find important. For example, the experience of contemplativeness and stillness might be more important to someone than stimulation and busyness. Indeed, one of the co-authors (RB) recalls a man in a day care centre telling her how he would prefer to sit and read rather than make bird boxes, which is what other men attending the day centre were doing, but he didn't sit and read because he felt it was not the thing to do. He said, "that won't get me anywhere, will it". In order to move the debate towards social citizenship it is necessary to think beyond the psychosocial and therapeutic value of occupation and to think in a more citizen-focused way about what might be purposeful and meaningful.

People with dementia do not talk of needing occupation, but they do talk about needing a purpose and meaning in life (see, for example, Taylor, 2009). In addition, clinical psychologist Steve Sabat (2002, p 6) describes a poignant moment for him in his career when a man with Alzheimer's disease, while undergoing a series of tests, said to him, "Doc, you've gotta find a way to give us *purpose* again" (emphasis added). This man was not expressing a need for occupation, but rather purpose – a reason to be in the world. Similarly, Terry Pratchett has made it clear how he plans to continue writing novels for as long as he can – presumably because he regards writing novels as his main purpose in life. It is important that the field works from a framework built on the narratives of people with dementia, rather than disciplinary knowledge. This means using the language of purpose, not occupation, and recognising that this may differ at the individual level. A person might derive meaning and a sense of purpose from a practical activity, like making bird boxes, but they might not.

From inclusion to participation

The importance of inclusion for people with dementia is well established. In particular, the inclusion of people with dementia in decisions about their care is increasingly promoted and practiced. The notion of inclusion is given extra weight when conceptualised alongside the notion of a 'sense of significance', as this stresses how a person's involvement and contributions to everyday life must be recognised and valued (Ryan et al, 2008, p 81). Thus it is not enough to simply include people in decisions about their care; we must also convey to the person that their inclusion matters.

However, there are three issues related to how the notion of inclusion has been developed to date that render it potentially problematic. First, too frequently it has been used narrowly to reference a person's role within their care environment. This has led to new and innovative care practices while potentially limiting the breadth and range of opportunities afforded to people with dementia. It is important to extend conceptualisations still further and consider the broader spectrum of social activities and processes that people with dementia have a right to or might wish to participate in. These might include, for example:

- remaining involved in the local theatre group
- continuing to work in their chosen occupation
- developing media responses to educate others about dementia
- serving on relevant boards and committees
- participating in adult continuing educational programmes
- voting in local and national elections.

This range of activities begins to hint at the second constraint of inclusion. That is, that it tends to imply mere presence rather than activity: the passivity of the word 'inclusion' is problematic. Acting, working, learning, voting ... these are actions – more than just inclusion; people with dementia have the right to *participate* in their lives at whatever level they can.

Participation is a more active verb that recognises that people with dementia have agency, that is, they seek self-control and act in a way that has subjective meaning. The link between participation and citizen control has long been recognised (Arnstein, 1969); however, it is only recently that the idea has been debated in the context of people with dementia. For example, Cantley et al (2005) use the notion of citizen participation to outline a range of activities that people with dementia can, and do, participate in, including, for example, making their views known about the activities they would like to see in a care setting, influencing the way an organisation provides care, contributing to community-based events and national groups, and participating in global organisations like DASNI and Alzheimer's Disease International (ADI). Clearly, the scope for genuine participation is increasing and the importance of involving people as active citizens is recognised.

However, even here, citizen participation is only discussed and applied in the context of dementia-related issues and services; there remains a lack of consideration of the participation of people with dementia in wider sociopolitical systems and debates. Like the field of older people services generally, there is a tendency within dementia care to think only in terms of people's participation as consumers of health/social care services (Scourfield, 2007). Wider democratic processes and debates that people with dementia are entitled (and may wish) to participate in are overlooked or not properly considered.

This brings us to the third issue. Discussions of dementia and participation often invariably end up in discussions about incapacity. For example, with the diagnosis of dementia, there has often been an assumption that a person can, or should, no longer participate in decision making at governmental level because the diagnosis is implicitly associated with assumed incapability. The reality is that someone with early dementia may still want – and be able – to vote in governmental or other elections. Moreover, as long as the person 'understands the process and consequence of voting, and can choose candidates', they have an inalienable right, as a citizen, to do so (Wislowski, 2006, p 69). Similarly, someone with dementia may want to participate in debates or seek to influence policy decisions about issues unrelated to dementia care, for example, the environment, public transport, fuel poverty and so forth. However, because of pervasive fears linking dementia to incapacity, these issues have not been thoroughly explored or debated; hence a gap in knowledge remains about how best to assist people with this level and type of civic participation.

This is one area where legislative changes are leading the way in terms of a social citizenship approach. Specifically, at the international level new laws around guardianship, decision making and capacity are reasserting fundamental rights to the presumption of capacity and, in situations of incapacity, are mandating more refined understandings that seek to link the designation of incapacity to a specific decision. Furthermore, legislation like England's 2005 Mental Capacity Act expects that even those found incapable of making personal decisions will nevertheless *participate* in these decisions (Boyle, 2008). Participation, not simply inclusion, is increasingly recognised worldwide as a fundamental right and guiding principle in frameworks for health and ageing: people with dementia should be no exception.

There are three points related to the need to move beyond inclusion to consider participation. First, we need to consider the involvement of people with dementia in their own lives and decisions in a much more active way than notions of 'inclusion' encourage us to think. Second, conceptualisations about inclusion need to be extended to take account of a person's participation in a much broader range of decisions and debates than has previously been considered. Third, the notion of participation must recognise people's diverse abilities and that individual participation will look different depending on retained abilities, personal histories and opportunities. Extending the continuum of concepts from inclusion to participation helps to reframe that debate, and most importantly, reaffirms people's rights to actively participate in the communities, towns and cities in which they live.

From attachment to solidarity

In recent years, the psychological concept of attachment has proved extremely useful for enhancing understanding of the individual needs of people with dementia. Attachment can be defined as an emotional bond to another person. Psychologist John Bowlby (1907-90) was the first attachment theorist, describing attachment as a 'lasting psychological connectedness between human beings' (Bowlby, 1979, p 194). Much has been written in both practice journals and academic literature about the importance of a person with dementia being able to feel a sense of attachment to someone or something, even if this is just a doll or a pet (for a useful summary of attachment theory and the literature on attachment in dementia care see, for example, Miesen, 2006).

While the concept of attachment is clearly important, using it indiscriminately and universally in all discourse about people with dementia is problematic. One problem with the idea of attachment is that it is essentially a submissive one; it assumes a person with dementia psychologically connects with something and that that 'something' is where the power and energy will lie. A second problem is that it seeks to explain actions and experiences in purely emotional terms, that is, as a 'psychological connectedness'. No account is taken of broader sociopolitical relations – such as the new forms of activism by people with dementia discussed at the start of this book – or the connections and responsibilities a person with dementia might feel towards other people with dementia. Actions that help wider society are critical for social citizenship but they remain outside the lens when the idea of attachment is the only one used to analyse the connections a person has or needs.

In cognate disciplines, such as citizenship studies, disability studies, social and urban policy, the concept of solidarity is increasingly used to move forward the debate about social citizenship. Solidarity is defined in these debates as uniting with others to make a difference; thus, unlike attachment, this idea is concerned with the shape of society as a whole, as well as the individual needs of citizens. The notion of solidarity is based on the belief that in order for society to progress, it needs people to get together and to take some form of united action (Thake, 2008). An obvious example of how this is happening in the field of dementia studies is, of course, with the proliferation of campaign groups like DASNI and SDWG, but it is important to also think of solidarity in relation to more everyday practices. Take for instance the way in which a small group of men with dementia in a long-term care facility might form an alliance – go round with each other – in order to perhaps counter the feminised aspects of that society (Bartlett, 2007); or how younger people with dementia have united to form their own peer support groups. While the ideas of attachment might explain how such actions address a person's need for 'psychological connectedness', it does not explain the difference such actions can make to the local community as a whole. The idea of solidarity can; it apprehends that some people can and will want to take responsibility for others, and that certain individuals connect with each other on a political, as well as emotional level.

From love to freedom from discrimination

According to Kitwood (1997a), a central need for people with dementia is love. People need to feel cared for, cherished, and above all, respected. This was, and still is, an important message for not only the health and social care field, but also society more generally. In recent years this message has given rise to a greater concern in both practice and research for the emotional needs of people with dementia. For example, Rewston and Moniz-Cook (2008) discuss ways of alleviating emotional distress for people with dementia.

However, while the notion of love is clearly an important one for the field of dementia care, it may not always be the most appropriate or effective one for bringing about change, particularly when 'love' actually manifests as control. From a critical disability perspective, the 'cosy image of care as synonymous with love can serve to mask the control that operates in many relationships where one person is substantially dependant on another' (Swain et al, 2003, p 142). With this view, we must consider how even in the most loving of relationships or care environments an individual's rights and entitlements can be easily undermined or curtailed. Think, for example, of how controlling and overwhelming some 'loving' family members can be. Also think how effectively residents living in a long-term care facility can be controlled from making too many demands – and hence having their needs met – due to their concerns about burdening overworked, stressed care workers. Clearly, the language of love – or care – is ineffectual when it comes to conceptualising the broader discriminatory experiences that people with dementia continue to face.

People with dementia are entitled to experience freedom from discrimination as well as love. The right to be free from negative discrimination is central to citizenship. People with dementia can be discriminated against at a macro and micro level. On a macro level, people with dementia can be discriminated against in the sense that they are denied access to certain services or benefits. For example, in the UK, because of the way mobility constraints are defined, people affected by dementia cannot apply for a blue badge[1] (Social Exclusion Unit, 2006, p 94). On a micro level, people with dementia are discriminated against every time someone assumes that because they have a diagnosis of dementia, they cannot speak on their own behalf. The main effect of discrimination against people with dementia, at whatever level, is that it compounds the neurological-related problems a person already has and reduces opportunities for self-expression and growth (Woods, 2001). It is for these reasons that discrimination is recognised as a public health issue (Link and Phelan, 2006). The freer people with dementia are from discrimination the more likely their status in society will improve. The language of love and care is neither sufficiently powerful nor critical enough to address these contradictions and issues.

Conclusion

This chapter has sought to analyse the concept of citizenship from the perspective of people with dementia and to posit an understanding of it that is workable for dementia studies. Some of the ideas in this chapter may seem radical or difficult to grasp at the moment but in 10 years' time we believe they are likely to be less so. As the number of activists with dementia increases, and a new generation of people with dementia begin to use services and complain about poor practice and the discrimination they face, we expect that thinking about and using the concept of citizenship will become more commonplace.

The conceptual framework presented in this chapter is designed to facilitate and support such expansions in thinking and practice. The reason for extending the continuum of concepts is to (re)position the person with dementia as an active agent with rights and a fluid or semi-degree of responsibility. In addition, the goal is to provide a language for taking a critical perspective, which is urgently required from the field.

Note

[1] Blue badges provide parking concessions to people with certain disabilities.

Part II
Social citizenship in action

FOUR

Thinking and talking differently

Introduction

While ideas associated with a social citizenship approach to practice may be conceptually intriguing, their real value lies in their potential to inform practice. In this chapter we argue that the first step in changing practice is to become more aware of the ways that we support and/or inadvertently sabotage the realisation of a critical social citizenship in people with dementia. Thus, the purpose of this chapter is to begin to demonstrate how analysing the situation of people with dementia from a sociopolitical perspective rooted in social theories of lifecourse, disability and citizenship can change the way we think about people with dementia. This includes challenging our own attitudes, beliefs and values about their rights and issues.

In order to frame this discussion we will draw on the ideas of post-structuralism to examine the power of language for constructing how we think and act. The main idea posited here is that at a very general level our understandings and actions are informed and shaped by the language that is available to us for making sense. Following a brief overview of the rationale behind this statement, we will then identify some of the problematic and limiting ways that language is implicitly used to understand dementia experiences. We highlight the need to begin to explicitly interrogate how we use language to tease out the underlying assumptions, values and beliefs that are guiding how we understand and interact with people who have dementia. Alternative ways for reframing and using language differently, to draw on ideas more consistent with a critical social citizenship approach, are then discussed.

Power of language

> "The more familiar they are with me, I feel more at ease. You know, if they want to call me [by my first name] Annie, fine. But … there are only a certain type of people that insist on that." (older woman living with dementia in a residential care setting)

In a small study comparing the experiences of residents with dementia living in a long-term care facility to those without dementia conducted by one of the authors (DO), one of the striking differences that began to emerge was the importance that those with dementia placed on how they were named. They differed in what their preferences were – for example, one spoke with pleasure about the staff calling her 'mama' while another participant expressed outrage at being called anything but 'Mrs [Surname]'. To Annie, the participant above, it was important that she was called by her first name, as this denoted a familiarity that she found comforting. While participants differed in *what* their preferences were, the notable observation was that most *did* express a preference related to how they were referenced and provided some rationale behind this choice. In some way, all recognised this seemingly minor exchange as one way that staff conveyed to them their position within the facility. Thus, at a micro level, the responses of these older adults reflect the importance of language, in this case naming, as a means for constructing personal experiences.

Language does not just influence how we understand ourselves and others. Rather, drawing on the ideas of post-structuralism, there is growing recognition of the importance of language for shaping experience at a broader, societal level as well. Post-structuralism, referenced by some as postmodernism,[1] describes an intellectual and cultural movement that shifts the focus from a notion of pre-existing, stable reality to the importance of language for constructing reality. In other words, 'reality' is not out there as some impermeable, fixed state, but instead it is constructed through and by our use of language. An important notion underpinning this understanding is that language is not neutral. Rather, it is linked to particular 'discourses', a term that refers to interrelated systems of statements which cohere around common meanings and reflect sets of assumptions, values and beliefs that are socially shared. Discourses – also referred to as a storyline (Davis, 2002) – provide abstract guidelines or parameters on which individuals draw to make sense of the world and their own personal experiences. At any given time, there are multiple discourses – or storylines – available that can be used for meaning making. These can complement one another or compete to create distinct and incompatible versions of reality. However, while there are diverse storylines or discourses, not all are of equal importance. Some have a privileged and dominant influence on language, thought and action. These are the discourses that impress as 'common sense'. They can often be recognised by the implicit 'should' that is used to guide personal actions and meaning making; for example, families 'should' take care of their frail elder relatives. An important point to remember is that discourses are not neutral; they represent political interests and are constantly vying for status and power (Weedon, 1987, p 41).

At a practical level, discourses can be identified through the language being used, both in day-to-day conversation but also in documents such as public policy statements and practice procedures. Put another way, the language we use – both oral and written – reflects systems of assumptions, values and beliefs. We may not be aware of the storylines on which we are drawing, and we may not be attuned to how these are being used to guide our actions and meaning making, but they are nonetheless shaping our attitudes, as well as our personal and interpersonal interactions. For example, drawing again on the storyline that families *should* care for their frail elder relatives means that someone *will* feel guilty about institutionalising their relative because they are not performing as they 'should'.

Recognising the importance of language for constructing reality offers an important route for reflecting on personal practices and can lead to challenging those that are potentially oppressive or problematic. This creates new possibilities. Specifically, if language constructs reality, the exciting promise is that reality can be changed by changing our language. This means that questioning and taking apart the language and words that we use to think about a situation is one way of identifying hidden problematic ideas that may be informing our attitudes and responses in a given situation; consciously changing our language can lead to developing new 'realities' that may be more relevant and productive.

Within the field of dementia studies there has been some recognition of the importance of language for constructing the experience in a particular way. For example, in the move towards a more humanistic lens, a shift in language from the dementia 'victim' or 'patient' to the 'person with dementia' is purposeful to counter the reductionism affiliated with the biomedical lens (which arguably constitutes a dominant discourse in dementia studies). More recently, people with dementia themselves have begun to lay claim to how language is used to describe their experiences. For example, the use of 'dementia' is now being publicly criticised not only for its reductionism and assumptions about 'normal/ abnormal cognitive functioning' (see, for example, Hachinski, 2008) but also for its problematic alignment with the notion of madness (for a discussion of this issue see, for example, Trachtenberg and Trojanowski, 2008). Similarly, others with dementia have laid claim to the acronym PWD (person with dementia) as a preferred means of self-identification (Lynn Jackson, personal communication).

Unfortunately, despite the above example, too frequently the discussion around language has occurred at the conceptual level; the translation into professional practice or public discourse has often lagged behind. Moreover, the focus on language has not always been taken far enough, and as identified in earlier chapters, cracks in new ways of using language are beginning to emerge in relation to how they position people with dementia. This is to be expected – all language will promote some realities while masking, or marginalising, others.

The remainder of this chapter will examine how language can be used to think about and inform practices that are more congruent with a social citizenship lens. It will be organised around two main activities:

- deconstructing discourse: interrogating personal assumptions, values and beliefs
- restructuring a framework: using language strategically and deliberately.

Deconstructing discourse: interrogating personal assumptions, values and beliefs

Oppressive and discriminatory practices often have their foothold in the well-meaning, well-intentioned ideas of those least intending to do harm. Arguably, few individuals would knowingly suggest that people with dementia no longer count as 'real' people with real rights. Still fewer would suggest that we as a society 'should' turn these individuals into 'non-people'. And yet, as the work of Kitwood and others began to make explicit, this is often an unintended consequence of talking about the lives of people with dementia in a particular way. This body of work highlighted the importance of shifting from a purely biomedical discourse to a more humanistic one by initiating a closer scrutiny of the assumptions, values and beliefs that were being used to ground understanding of the experiences of people with dementia when the biomedical lens was used exclusively. These reflections led to clearer standing and status for people with dementia, an important step towards recognising social citizenship.

So to avoid unintentionally using ideas that may be oppressive, the importance of intentionally beginning to deconstruct someone's personal systems of assumptions, values and beliefs emerges as a critical starting point to practice. When we deconstruct, ways of understanding the world are not accepted as givens but rather examined and interrogated in relation to their social, historical and political contexts. This interrogation requires directing attention to the excluded and marginal because 'it is through this process that seemingly smooth social surfaces and accepted wisdom can be disrupted and the space created for alternative discourses' (Opie, 2000, p 23). Deconstructing personal assumptions, values and beliefs is the core of reflexive practice.

The first step in this process of critical reflection is to identify the storylines that are being used to frame someone's personal meaning making. This includes recognising the likelihood that multiple storylines may be used simultaneously and that these storylines may support one another but may also create tensions because they result in competing and incompatible versions of reality. For example, we can firmly believe that people with dementia have the right to societal support while simultaneously holding the perspective that family members should care for their relatives with dementia. Both are good ideas but there are points where they contradict one another. The implication of this is to expect that we can rarely rely on having *one* coherent frame of reference – what we consciously think we are promoting may be undermined by less consciously recognised frames of reference.

Part of the process of identifying the storylines that are being used to frame personal meaning is to recognise that these reflect cultural interpretations and understandings. There is no such thing as a universal discourse. Rather, we all have our own cultural baggage that we draw on – either consciously or sub-consciously – to inform how we make sense of the world. Problems emerge when we assume that our way of understanding is the 'only' way of understanding.

Thus, a second step in this process is to open these storylines up to critical questioning in order to make visible what assumptions, values and beliefs are underpinning each. For instance, what are the assumptions underpinning discussions about 'managing challenging behaviours' when discussing the situation of someone with dementia? Are these assumptions acceptable to you? Part of this process is attending to points of discomfort and tension – these help make visible the taken-for-granted dominant discourses that, as noted above, can often be identified by the implicit 'shoulds' that often leave you feeling guilty or inadequate.

Again, returning to the notion of family care, with little hesitancy most would sanction it. However, as many feminists have pointed out, too often family care is accepted with little attention given to its negative possibilities. These negative possibilities become clearer only when scrutinised more critically. One implication, for example, is that it implicitly places familial relationship above the personal qualities, skills and capabilities required for providing good care and leaves family members feeling guilty and deficient when they are not able to provide care, even when the caring situation has clearly surpassed their personal skill level.

> Mr Green is a 76-year-old married man who was identified as the primary caregiver for his wife who had dementia. He agreed to participate in a research study exploring the experiences of living with a partner who had dementia. During an exploratory interview with him, he made clear that he felt like a "prisoner" and would gladly relinquish the care of his wife except for the knowledge that he would "cease to have sons" should he not do his duty. He described himself as an impatient man with exacting standards for himself and others and noted that these personal characteristics had served him well as a businessman but were not conducive to effective caregiving. He could not understand how people could expect him to change overnight and suddenly become a loving, patient man when this simply wasn't his nature. He identified his desire for a sexual relationship and expressed his bitterness that his wife's illness prevented him from attending to his own needs.
>
> What a selfish, thoroughly dislikeable man, I [DO] thought as I drove away. Later, surprised by the intensity and judgemental quality of my reaction, I began to reflect upon my response. I realised that I was offended by Mr Green because his words had challenged the dominant notion of 'family care' – a storyline that I obviously had bought into without even realising it.

By locating the family care storyline as preferred, other types of caring, including care by formal caregivers and/or institutionalisation, by default are positioned as inferior. This storyline works to the advantage of policy makers who save money in healthcare through the efforts of family members. However, it can have unintended effects, including pressuring family members into taking on caring responsibilities for which they are ill suited. Furthermore, it can unintentionally undermine social citizenship by positioning family carers to speak on the person's behalf; historically, there has been a tendency to accord family members higher credibility and responsibility around decision making, irrespective of whether this is warranted or not. The notion of family care can therefore indirectly result in the positioning of the person with dementia as a care recipient, silencing him/her and eroding his/her rights to full social citizenship. It can also render invisible those who have no family.

Virginia lives alone with dementia and was motivated to volunteer to participate in a study exploring how people with dementia and their family interacted with formal support services largely because she felt she had "something important" to say about the damage done when others implicitly assumed the presence of a supportive family. Her story of living with dementia centred round what she clearly described as ultimately "a journey I had to take myself". This journey is made more difficult because of the failure of others to realise that she is on her own. Rather, because she has two sons and a daughter – two of whom are geographically within reasonable commuting distance including a son who lives in her neighbourhood – "everyone" assumes they are there to help her. However, for various reasons, including her wish not to burden two of her children who are going through their own personal crises – and their wish to keep it this way – and a strained relationship with her geographically closest son, her children are not a source of support. "And the people in my family, I mean forget it, when it comes to having family members involved some of them are fabulous, they seem to know instinctively when to encourage you to push on and when to, to encourage you to sit back, you know. That would be wonderful! But that wouldn't be my family – it's all very well for me to wish at times that I had this wonderful support system but I'm better off with what I've got even though I've gone through times when I was totally and utterly lost." She describes her anger, frustration and the sense of abandonment that occurred because those helping her made erroneous assumptions about the role of family in her life.

The intention behind drawing attention to this discourse is not to devalue family care, nor is it to suggest that family care is necessarily a problematic storyline. Rather, it is to recognise that it *can* be a potentially oppressive storyline when alternative realities are not permitted, or recognised. It *can* have unintended effects. Thus, it provides an example to highlight how important it is for health and social care practitioners to consciously scrutinise the values, beliefs and assumptions that they are intentionally, and/or unintentionally drawing on to ensure they are not inadvertently marginalising some people, especially those with dementia.

The above discourse is not unique in its hidden oppressive potential; all discourses, or storylines, have unintended repercussions. A similar contradiction emerges when storylines that depict the dementia experience as a deteriorating biomedical condition are pitted against the notion of social citizenship in dementia. Individually, both 'storylines' have credibility and most health and social care practitioners would give a nod of approval to the assumptions underpinning both. Yet one contradiction that is beginning to emerge regards the delicate balance a person with dementia has to maintain in terms of showing themselves to be articulate and mindful (like Lynn Jackson and Richard Taylor) without jeopardising their 'status' as someone with dementia: people who 'look too good' or do not conform to normative ways of progressing through the dementia may end up having their credibility challenged as someone who doesn't *really* have dementia.

Moreover, the needs they do have as a result of neuropathological changes may be overlooked. Virginia, a 69-year-old woman with multi-infarct dementia, who struggles to retain her independence and autonomy, describes how this is used against her:

> "I mean I have a son, he's told his wife there's nothing wrong with me, physically, dementia wise.... I am looking for attention. That was so painful – I suspected it, but it was so painful to hear that. It's just and so they see you on your good days and they think you're fine, you're okay, but I tell people who say you always seem to do everything so well and I'll say because you don't see me on my bad days, I stay home, I don't go out, I don't communicate with people because I don't, I can't, you know, or it's so much work, I just don't feel up to it so I don't go out, you know."

Similarly, Betty, an aboriginal woman who drew on her cultural ancestry and value base to see the diagnosis of dementia as an opportunity for growth and development, repeatedly described how others, including her physician and family, constantly undermined the severity of her symptoms and the difficulties she was encountering because she failed to conform to the medicalised understanding of dementia as loss and deterioration. At one point this resulted in her disability pension being revoked (see O'Connor et al, 2009). A theme underpinning both of these women's stories is the double-bind that each felt as the work they did to use the diagnosis constructively led others to misinterpret, challenge or negate the difficulties they were experiencing. It is a theme that is similarly raised throughout Richard Taylor's monthly chronicles about his experiences as a politically active person with dementia (see, for example, the June 2009 newsletter at www.richardtaylorphd.com).

The point here is twofold. First, old ways of understanding are deeply embedded and without realising it – and even in light of explicitly articulated alternative viewpoints – we may unintentionally draw on storylines that are problematic. Second, different storylines can result in confusing pictures with inherent contradictions that need to be acknowledged and untangled to prevent inadvertently perpetrating oppressive practices. In other words, reflexive practice demands that we continuously scrutinise how we are making meaning and how this implicates our actions. All storylines must be open to critical interrogation. This, then, is a starting point towards a more sociopolitical approach to dementia. It is through this process of opening up to interrogation the storylines that they are using, that health and social care workers can begin to examine the ways that they 'contribute to social control by subtly holding clients in powerless positions and reinforcing identities ascribed to them by the dominant order' (Fook, 1993).

Some questions that can help guide this reflexive interrogation include the following:

- What are the 'storylines' that you are drawing on to make sense of this person's experiences? What are the underlying assumptions, values and beliefs being used to construct these storylines?
- How do different storylines support and/or contradict one another?
- What possibilities are being excluded when a particular storyline is taken up as the preferred reality? In particular, what storylines foster inclusive social citizenship for people with dementia and their family? Which ones challenge it?
- Whose voices are being heard? Whose voices are being silenced?

Restructuring a framework: using language strategically and deliberately

If language constructs reality then attending to the use of language raises exciting possibilities for changing reality. Deconstructing, or critically interrogating personal assumptions, values and beliefs, begins the process of creating the space for change to occur. Often this process begins by attending to the language we use to think, talk and write about situations and experiences.

Finding new ways to use language strategically and deliberately is the means towards realising the possibility of change. This section explores the strategic use of language – oral and written, verbal and non-verbal – in order to promote practices that reflect different worldviews that are more congruent with a critical social citizenship approach to practice. It draws on the literature in this area and is organised around three overlapping and interrelated sub-themes: confronting 'othering' strategies, negotiating the dual focus on care *and* social justice, and documentation as a tactical tool: writing as resistance. The objective is to move beyond academic debates in order to link these ideas explicitly to practice.

Confronting 'othering' strategies

Language is an effective tool for 'othering'. In its most basic form the use of a 'we' and 'they' establishes boundaries that position the other – the 'they' – as not like us. This is problematic because it sets up categories of belonging that only account for one aspect of identity, an identity that is based on difference. Kitwood's work first drew attention to this, highlighting that positioning people only in relation to whether or not they had dementia tended to obliterate all other aspects of that person (for a comprehensive discussion about this see also Steven Sabat's work: Sabat and Harre, 1992; Sabat, 2001, 2005). The shift from language focused on the 'patient' to considering the 'person with dementia' represents one move towards redressing this. However, people with dementia are still being positioned as 'other', as though the dementia experience is the only aspect of the person's identity that warrants attention. A growing body of literature critiques this tendency because it portrays dementia as a homogeneous, shared experience that negates all other aspects of a person's identity.

The struggle here, rarely confronted in the humanist literature but more widely discussed in relationship to critical social citizenship, is to recognise that people with dementia both belong to a particular 'cultural' group based on differing experiences (a diagnosis of dementia) *and* simultaneously see similarities with their own social membership. Lister (2007) articulates this as the tension between citizenship's inclusionary and exclusionary sides (Lister, 2007; see also Egeland and Gressgard, 2007, for a discussion of this issue). Reflecting the tensions between group politics and complexity, the challenge here is how to avoid essentialising the experience of dementia while simultaneously creating a common ground since it is through the development of this common ground that social action is possible. In other words, how do we ensure that there is both a 'they', or community of people with dementia, and a 'we' that diminishes the boundaries of othering?

Thus, on the one hand, recognising people with dementia as a cultural group is important because a sense of solidarity is a priority for political mobilisation and social action to occur and different needs to be recognised in order to respond appropriately. Skeggs (2004, p 38), for example, identifies the importance of providing 'a rhetorical space where the experiences and knowledge of the marginalized can be given epistemic authority, be legitimated and taken seriously'. On the other hand, people's positioning is relational and context specific: this is reflected in a letter by Jim Mann to his MP, where he positions himself not only as a social advocate and person with dementia but also a family member caring for an ageing mother. Another woman with dementia similarly articulates this need to be seen both with dementia but also beyond the dementia:

> "And it's my experience with everything that's been happening with me, it's, it's multifaceted and people have a tendency to forget, we don't just have dementia, we have other issues happening, we have family issues happening or we have physical things happening and they all influence each other."

Thus, while the struggle for inclusion has been an important part of the shift towards a citizenship lens, the challenge is to formulate this concept from the standpoint of those with dementia while avoiding the tendency to categorise people with dementia only as 'different'.

This is a complicated issue and it remains unclear how best to address it. Consciously using language that reflects fluid ways of positioning is a start. This means that health and social care practitioners need to learn to speak of people with dementia both as a 'we' and as a 'they' depending on context; it is through our use of language that we position others. It also means that this positioning must be done in ways that are both dynamic and strategic. McCall (2005) believes this can be achieved by the 'provisional adoption' of organising categories depending on context. This requires recognising multiple identities but prioritising some over others depending on context as defined by the end goal. For example, sometimes it is important to speak of 'people with dementia' in order to achieve a coherent sociopolitical context with group members. At other times, the language of 'people with dementia' may be more appropriate because it allows for both the plurality but also the contextualised individuality to be more visible. Still other times, it may be more appropriate to speak of a 'we' since it is all of us who are penalised by our 'hypercognitive society' (Post, 2000). Similarly, it may serve a useful purpose to talk about 'service users' and 'family carers' or 'caregivers' at particular points, but to 'see' people solely within these categories is problematic.

The point here is to highlight the importance of referential language as one tactic for creating inclusionary, and exclusionary, citizenships. How we reference others both vis-à-vis ourselves and in relation to particular categories has important implications. It can lead to unintentionally 'othering' people with dementia (and carers), which can in turn result in wiping out aspects of personal identity, indirectly fostering a storyline that people with dementia can *only* be understood as 'people with dementia', and carers can *only* be understood as 'carers'.

Reflexive questions to promote thinking about 'othering' include:

- How is the person with dementia being positioned? How is my use of language reinforcing this positioning?
- What is achieved through this positioning?
- (How) does this positioning limit the person with dementia?
- (How) does this positioning elevate their status?
- How is language being used to achieve this positioning?

Negotiating the dual focus on care and social justice

Discussions about the dementia experience are invariably cushioned within the language of 'caring' or 'supporting'. This is both informally through conversations and formally in the form of written care plans, policies and guidelines. While this language is undoubtedly appropriate in certain contexts, the danger with it is that it can denote a one-way relationship that permanently positions the person with dementia only as someone who needs to be taken care of. There are two issues here. First, it fails to recognise the contributions that people with this diagnosis can make both in interpersonal relationships and to society in general. This includes both within the caring relationship but also within other types of relationships, such as that of a friend or neighbour. Second, it positions dependence as a static position that is necessarily inferior and in opposition to independence (to be discussed in more detail later). These implications are counter to a social citizenship lens.

The dual focus between social justice and care has been recognised as a 'tightrope' that is complicated to traverse (Barnes and Brannelly, 2008). It is generally accepted that at some point many people with dementia will require 'care' and social justice arguments related to notions of rights and responsibilities can be critiqued for failing to value dependency and caring as part of normative relational connections. For example, Kittay (1999) argues that the myth of independence is damaging to the pursuit of political and social practices that embody an understanding of inequality, but which are also compatible with the demands of fairness and connection. She highlights the importance of considering the circumstances of those who are most dependent and of those who care for them, in order to explore ways in which social responsibility is exercised, arguing that starting from assumptions of equality will not lead to policies and practices that will meet the requirements of 'justice for all' (Kittay, 1999, p xiii).

Feminists have been particularly vocal about calling for a relational ethics of care that challenges the prioritising of the independent, autonomous being and instead values interdependencies, connections and relational vulnerabilities (see, for example, Sherwin, 1992). The challenge becomes to determine how a relational ethics of care can be incorporated into a social justice lens. For example, Barnes and Brannelly (2008, p 394) argue that an ethics of practice and social justice cannot be achieved on the basis of a series of moral principles, but neither is an exclusively rights-based approach adequate to ensure justice when people occupy very different positions in terms of their need for help.

While these debates have been ongoing, they have largely happened at an abstract, conceptual level. However, they translate into significant implications at the practice level. If people with dementia are to be recognised as both active agents *and* as people who may require additional support and care at some point in their journey, then a continuum of responses must be recognised and new language developed that reflects the fluid statuses of people with dementia without valorising some positions over others.

One way of negotiating these dual foci is to find ways to bridge oppositional language. As a society we have often used language to create boundaries and categories: things are defined in relation to what they are not, creating the impression that they are mutually exclusive and that this dichotomy captures the only possibilities. There are several areas where these occur in the field of dementia that challenge a dual focus on care and citizenship.

The notion of dependency represents one of the most common ways that a boundary is accomplished within the field of dementia. Here, the notion of dependency is pitted against the notion of independence, with independence always being that accorded higher value. Within disability studies, one means towards challenging the simplicity of this oppositional language has been to refocus on the concept of *interdependency*. It is important because it recognises that even in situations where someone may be profoundly dependent on another person to have his/her care needs met, that supporting person is still often getting something out of the relationship. Unfortunately, with few exceptions, this notion has rarely been extended to examine the relationship between those with dementia and the people caring for them. Using the language of interdependence to write, think and talk about the situations of people with dementia then, brings to the forefront the importance of asking a different set of questions when considering a particular situation. For example, what is the family member getting from his/her relationship with the person with dementia? How is the person with dementia contributing to his or her social milieu?

Another example where oppositional language is often apparent in dementia studies is in the tendency to compartmentalise people as either caregivers/carers or care receivers. Again, the use of this language creates the impression that one can be one or the other, but not both. It also reduces the complexity of mutuality in a relationship by prioritising one aspect of giving care – usually that of physical care – and ignoring that a person can give care and still receive care, albeit perhaps in a different format. Research is accumulating to suggest that this is both too simplistic and inaccurate (see, for example, O'Connor, 1995; O'Connor et al, 2007; Davis and Nolan, 2008). Reflecting the move towards more dynamic, relational understandings, shifting language to talk about 'care partners' has been one way that this artificial dichotomising has been addressed.

The point here is to recognise that health and social care practitioners can introduce new ways of describing and talking that challenge the positioning of the person with dementia as only someone who requires care and is dependent on others. In doing so, they begin to create the space for social citizenship to become more visible.

A second way for strategically using language to accommodate the focus on care and social justice has been through experimenting with reconceptualising core concepts related to care. Barnes and Brannelly (2008), for example, redefine care:

> Care includes both self-care and care for others: It does not oppose dependence and independence but recognizes that we are all givers and receivers of care at different times; it is not linked to gender or "women's work"; it acknowledges bodily, spiritual and material aspects, the perspectives of caregivers and care-receivers, the existence of power and conflict within care, and the moral dimension of care. (p 203)

This definition normalises the notion of care and removes some of the pejorative connotations that can be associated with the concept. It fails, however, to recognise that as dementia progresses there may be points where much mutuality is either lost and/or harder to locate. Thus, while the person providing support may be getting something out of the care relationship – as recognised in relational approaches – it would be a disservice to family members and formal caregivers to discount the growing imbalance in the relationship that will undoubtedly occur as the dementia progresses. Hence, while attempting to reconceptualise core concepts around care represents an important step forward, further grappling with the language is still needed in order to avoid perpetuating an understanding and way of thinking that is still flawed.

A third way of addressing this dichotomy is to begin to recognise the notion of care as a continuum and to find language that reflects this. One way that this is happening is that new language is beginning to emerge that recognises the possibility that health and social care professionals can learn from people with dementia and family carers. For example, in Canada, there is a growing focus on 'knowledge exchange' as a two-way process that can facilitate meaningful dialogue between service users and providers. This notion recognises that health and social care professionals have something to offer people with dementia and their family, but also that people with dementia and their families have something to teach health and social care professionals. The intent is to demonstrate that by shifting the language of 'support' to that of 'exchange', implicitly the person with dementia and family carers are positioned as more equal contributors. This may then begin to place the involvement of people with dementia along a continuum – from that of advocate and health promotion to someone requiring more extensive support and care. Further, it reflects the notion that particularly in the advent of new medications and earlier diagnosis, people may have many years where they are defined less by their health and social care 'needs' and more by their unique insights and capacity to influence the system, thus moving us towards a more humane and just society.

A fourth strategic use of language to negotiate the balance between care and citizenship is to begin to purposefully incorporate stronger action words into practice. Expressions such as 'personhood' and 'person-centred' might be intuitively appealing and are certainly required to ground understanding and practice, but they also lead to individualised needs-based language that underpins notions of caring. On the other hand, 'rights-based talk' implicitly repositions the person with dementia as a citizen. Words such as 'entitlement, 'fairness' and 'justice' move away from the notion that people are asking for something for which they need to be grateful, and move instead into an assumption of legitimacy and value. For example, O'Connor (1999) found that when spouses living with a partner who had dementia could frame the use of services as a legitimate right, they were better able to successfully use support services. One participant from this study provides insight into this:

> Alice Cook cared for her mother in the community for several years before finally having her admitted into a care facility. She described how vital the community supports had been in helping her to successfully maintain her mother in the community for such a long time. Yet, despite her positive experiences with these services, two years later she was emaciated, depressed and in poor health as she struggled to meet her husband's care needs independently, adamantly refusing to take advantage of any of the community supports that were available to her. When asked how she accounted for her different responses to the use of services, Mrs Cook noted that as a daughter caring for her mother she recognised that she was entitled to some support since her primary allegiance had to be to her husband. However, she felt

caring for her husband was a wife's duty, and *needing* help with this would mean that she was not doing a very good job. (emphasis added).

In summary, the point of this section has been to highlight the tightrope that currently prevails between drawing on a social justice approach to dementia that underpins notions of citizenship and recognising that care can be an integral part of this experience. Changing language strategically can usefully begin to create new realities surrounding this dual focus. This includes consciously challenging the use of oppositional language that indirectly fosters this division, and strategically using language to implement different ways of thinking.

Documentation as a tactical tool: writing as resistance

There is a long-held belief that 'the pen is mightier than the sword', yet the power of the written word in practice often remains unexamined.

> May Fender is a 91-year-old woman with whom I [DO] had a longstanding professional relationship. This included facilitating her admission from the community into a long-term care facility. About three months after she moved into the facility, I was surprised to read in the chart that she had a diagnosis of dementia – I was not aware of any medical testing which would have resulted in this diagnosis. I was, however, very concerned that in the previous month she had begun to experience serious memory loss, disorientation and irritability. With further checking I was able to determine that this diagnosis had simply 'appeared' without benefit of any diagnostic testing. The issue was that her now apparent confused state was being ignored and relegated to the status of dementia. When the diagnosis was challenged, further medical investigation did take place revealing kidney failure and drug toxicity. However, four months later, the diagnostic label of dementia appeared once again on her chart, quoting the original – now disproved – written diagnosis.

This story demonstrates the power of the written word. Even though Miss Fender's diagnosis of dementia had been disproved, it could not be removed from the written records. The word continued to exert power. Gradually, Miss Fender was seen, and treated, as someone who had dementia irrespective of the lack of medical support for this 'diagnosis'. Eventually, she was moved onto the 'dementia' unit. Her story demonstrates how important documentation can be in creating a lasting construction of someone.

Knowing this opens up the importance and possibility of utilising documentation strategically. Specifically, the content and format of documentation can be used purposefully to construct the person in a particular manner:

Mrs Jonas placed an emergency telephone call to the community mental health team from whom she had been receiving treatment for the past several months for depression. She was in tears and indicated that she 'needed to talk to someone'. She indicated that she was feeling so hopeless that she had fleetingly considered taking all her medication so that she could 'leave it all behind' – strong religious beliefs prevented her from acting on this impulse though. A quick review of her chart identified her as a 70-year-old widow living alone in her own home with a diagnosis of early dementia. It indicated that she had a longstanding history of depression with the first episode occurring following the birth of her youngest child. This most recent episode began several months ago, shortly after her husband died. From the detailed description of her medication treatment, located at the front of the chart, it was clear that Mrs Jonas had been doing so well that a decrease in medication had taken place a week earlier.

With this information, Mrs Jonas's problems were constructed primarily as a medical issue. The interpretation of her current crisis was that she was relapsing due to the medication changes. Given her despair and thoughts of suicide, a decision was made to admit her to the psychiatric unit in order to monitor and readjust her medication.

However, retrospectively another story about Mrs Jonas's experience could have been written that was equally valid but largely absent in any documented form:

Mrs Jonas's deceased husband was a violent man who abused both her and her two daughters physically and emotionally until his sudden heart attack nine months ago. Both daughters are bitter about their upbringing. Her eldest daughter, who left home very early related to the abuse, lives several hundred miles away; she rarely sees her mother but does maintain periodic telephone contact and is available in times of crisis. The youngest daughter maintains a taut but involved relationship with Mrs Jonas. However, she works full time, lives about 30 minutes away and, after trying for years, is pregnant for the first time and experiencing complications. Normally she spends Saturday with her mother but because of her current health issues, she has not seen her mother for the past several weeks. This means that Mrs Jonas is alone all weekend, a state she finds extremely distressing but about which she will not complain for fear of being perceived as a burden or endangering her much anticipated grandchild. Mrs Jonas's only other involvement outside her home is through her participation in a Senior's Day programme. Initiated several months ago as part of her treatment plan, she attends Mondays and Wednesdays and Fridays and by all accounts is thriving in the programme. Her call to the mental health team occurred on a Thursday morning of a four-day long weekend; she was expecting to have no human contact until the following Wednesday. Interestingly, although the chart clearly documented all medication treatments, what it did *not* note was that Mrs Jonas' regular worker had been calling her almost daily for several months. Although these calls were very brief, Mrs Jonas later described how the calls made her feel as though someone cared. This worker had taken a brief leave and the replacement worker did not know about these calls, so no one from the team had been in contact with Mrs Jonas for almost two weeks.

This construction of Mrs Jonas's situation begins to move beyond the medical issues to encourage a different way of thinking about the situation and opens up alternative ways of responding. However, given the format of the chart, there was ample space to insert medical information, and minimal space (at the back of the binder) to provide non-medical information. This meant an alternative reading of the situation was not readily available at the point of crisis.

Given the importance of language for constructing reality, paperwork should not be viewed as a benign, inconsequential activity. Rather, the way in which a person's care records are written actively supports particular constructions of that person. Questions begin to emerge regarding why some understandings get written, while others are noticeably absent. Moreover, opportunities are identified for resisting some renditions of 'reality' by writing into existence alternative stories. This means that incorporating a social citizenship lens requires consciously examining how documentation is being used to perpetrate a particular lens that restricts full citizenship.

Edna Wright lives alone in the community. She has a diagnosis of dementia and, in the past two years, her son has been assuming increasing responsibility for overseeing her care needs including organising for meal delivery, grocery shopping and banking. When I [DO] arrived for a scheduled visit one sunny afternoon, I found her outside hanging up the curtains that she had washed that morning. She had forgotten about my visit. However, I noted that following our telephone conversation earlier that week to schedule the meeting, she had been able to accurately write my visit into the calendar hanging on her fridge door. I returned to my office, where I wrote up a progress note indicating how well Mrs Wright seemed to be doing. As I finished, an updated neuropsychological assessment was given to me. It concluded that Mrs Wright was in the moderate to advanced stages of dementia based on the score results of her MMSE and WAIS-R testing. How, I wondered, had I 'gotten it so wrong'? The recommendation was that she required immediate admission into a long-term care facility. Later, I realised where the differences lay – I had been focusing on what Mrs Wright could do – her strengths –

the testing had revealed what she couldn't do – her deficits. It is not surprising then that the neuropsychologist and I had such conflicting reports. And while the neuropsychological testing did reveal important deficits, it was revealing to note that despite her appalling test scores, Mrs Wright continued to live with relative safety in the community for an additional two years – even after her son began to disengage himself from overseeing her care.

The point here is to demonstrate that documents depict a story and the author has choices regarding how that story will be heard and interpreted. Choosing to ensure that a more holistic picture of the person with dementia is included facilitates a lens that moves beyond simple biomedical explanations. The second point, however, is that some ways of writing are accorded a higher status than others. In particular, standardised measurement tools are often valorised, holding sway in a way that 'talking' does not. As we will discuss in the next chapter, standardised, structured ways of interacting can in fact work against citizenship. Nonetheless, an important point here is to consciously recognise the power of standardised tools and to respond to the need to find ways in writing to counteract this power.

However, it is not only *what* gets written that is important. Rather, the organisation or format of documentation also tells a story. For example, when social history is buried at the back of the 'patient's chart' (as the chart is routinely referenced even in a care home) and medication regime is the first thing that the reader sees, a particular picture is being presented regarding what is important. Being attuned to this allows health and social care workers to begin to question and 'rewrite' some stories.

This entails examining written documentation to determine how oppressive or limiting storylines are being perpetrated. Some questions identified by Pare (2002) that can assist in this process include the following:

- What is the physical make-up of the document? What does it look and feel like? What sections are included? What is the sequence of sections and why?
- What is the purpose of the document? For example, why is it produced and for whom? How does it help with treatment decisions? How does it limit?
- What are the effects of the documentation? For example, what kinds of thinking does it encourage/discourage and what kinds of actions are encouraged or discouraged?
- Who reads the document? For example, is it only used by professionals or do clients also read it? If not, why not?
- Who has access to the document?

Assessing the status of documentation can help make explicit the discourses that are guiding understandings. Once named, these practices can be challenged. This may mean, for example, finding ways to include content that draws on a different understanding. It may also require finding ways for this content to be read. For example, non-medical notes that are handwritten and segregated at the back of the document visually suggests the marginalisation of this understanding. In contrast, intermingling these notes with those of other health professionals (including the physician) improves their visibility and creates a more holistic understanding. Through writing and documentation processes, existing realities may quietly yet effectively be subverted and redefined.

Conclusion

Drawing on a social citizenship lens requires writing, thinking and talking about practice and people with dementia differently. Attending to language – both spoken and written – offers an important starting point in this process. The purpose of this chapter has been to draw attention to the importance of language as both an opening for challenging existing ideas and as a means towards creating alternative ways of understanding. In terms of practice, the focus on language has important implications. In particular, it highlights the priority for those working or interacting in the field of dementia to consciously attend to their use of language, ensuring that words reflect assumptions, values and beliefs that are conducive to a social citizenship understanding. Thus, an important component of a social citizenship lens for practice is the need to critically reflect on language, since the ultimate goal is to challenge taken-for-granted ways of understanding dementia and interacting with people who have been diagnosed with it. The exciting point here is that if societal 'reality' is constructed by language, it can similarly be changed through use of language.

Note
[1] It is recognised that there are differences between post-structuralism and postmodernism but for the purposes of this chapter these will not be explored. Our intent in making the link between the two here is to pull out their similarities, not their differences.

FIVE

Implications for social and health care practices

Introduction

New ideas about social citizenship and dementia demand new forms of practice. In the previous chapter we drew on ideas associated with social constructionism to highlight the importance of considering how language is used to create understandings and to inform practice. We suggest that attending to the use of language is an important way for tuning into oppressive ideas and reshaping how we think about dementia in a way that is more congruent with a social citizenship lens. We argue that critical self-reflection is the first step towards a social citizenship approach to practice, and that attention to language provides an important entry point for this reflexive practice.

The purpose of this chapter is to move beyond thinking and begin to envision the *doing* of practice that is grounded in the ideas of a critical social citizenship approach. Specifically, we draw on the literature associated with critical[1] social and health care practice to examine how professional practice in the field of dementia can be reshaped to reflect a social citizenship approach. We will pay particular attention to direct, case-based practice, recognising that this is where the majority of those who have professional responsibility for supporting people with dementia work. Simultaneously, however, we will be trying to begin to break down the artificial dichotomy between case-based practice (often positioned as micro level practice) and more macro level practices such as community and social development.

This chapter is organised into two sections. The first clarifies and examines the general principles for a social citizenship approach to practice. The starting point and basis for discussion is the conceptual framework advanced in Chapter Three. Using this framework, four principles are outlined to help provide the bridge between concept and practice. The second section highlights three strategic approaches for realising these principles. Combined, the goal of the chapter is to broaden the debate around dementia practice by putting forward a value-based approach to practice that is more explicitly political and congruent with social citizenship.

Principles of a social citizenship approach to dementia practice

A person-centred approach to practice recognises that an important aspect of the dementia experience is the emphasis placed on maintaining personhood through the disease process. Practices grounded in a person-centred care approach include recognition of the importance of knowing the person, including his/her biographical history, creating an environment that maximises opportunities for inclusion and success and retaining respectful and dignified interactions (for a fuller discussion of this approach, see Brooker, 2004). Relationship-based care extends these ideas to explicitly highlight relationships as the fundamental means towards ensuring quality care that respects personhood; in doing so, this approach draws attention to the notion that relationships are dynamic and multidimensional (for a more complete discussion of this approach, see Davis and Nolan, 2008). A social citizenship approach to practice is congruent with *both* of these approaches but takes practice one step further to insert a more critical perspective that is attuned to issues of power, agency, marginalisation and disempowerment within a broader sociopolitical context in which dementia occurs. Hence, we note that the ideas presented in this chapter extend approaches labelled as person-centred and relationship-centred; they do not challenge them. Rather, we assume these ideas as necessary starting points and examine how to move beyond them into a more explicitly anti-oppressive, political practice.

A social citizenship approach to practice is grounded in certain principles. These are values which help to ensure a person's status and rights as an equal citizen are recognised and upheld; they also give rise to a much broader conceptualisation of people's capacity to participate, entitlements and potential. Drawing on the conceptual framework developed in Chapters Two and Three, we have identified four interrelated principles for guiding practice in a social citizenship approach to dementia. These principles cohere around the foundational premise that social citizenship practice requires a fundamental shift in onus for change from the person with dementia to society at large.

Principles underpinning a social citizenship approach:

- Active participation by people with dementia in their own lives, and society at large, must be maximised and valued.
- The potential for growth and positivity within the dementia experience must be recognised and promoted.
- Individual experiences and circumstances must be understood as inextricably connected to broader sociopolitical and cultural dynamics and structures.
- Solidarity between people with dementia, achieved through the fostering of a sense of 'we' and community building, is a realistic goal that must be nurtured.

Maximising and valuing participation

Everyone, including those with dementia, has the right and will expect to participate to the fullest extent possible in their own lives, the community surrounding them and society as a whole. This is more than mere 'inclusion'; it means active involvement. Of course, involvement will mean different things to different people; for example, as noted in Chapter Three, involvement might be as simple as raising a finger or a smile in relation to care preferences, or it might be as complex as voting or taking part in a public consultation exercise.

In a social citizenship approach, a person's ability to participate at some level is assumed irrespective of cognitive capacity. This stance is consistent with the international move away from considering mental capacity as a binary status (competent/not competent) to one which recognises that abilities are linked to specific decisions/actions; a person may not be able to contribute in a meaningful way to all aspects of his/her life and/or society-at-large but s/he is usually able to participate in some aspects. The principle of maximising and valuing participation requires finding ways to ensure that everyone with dementia has the opportunity to participate in a way that is meaningful and suitable for them, both in relation to decisions that are relevant to their own care but also in relation to other types of decisions. Cantley et al (2005) provide a useful and comprehensive discussion about how to promote the involvement of people with dementia in decisions about their care and service development. However, as the following example illustrates, ensuring participation sometimes requires marked creativity on the part of others:

> In an attempt to incorporate more person-centred care processes, Sunnyvale nursing home decided to restructure their weekly team meetings to include the resident they were discussing in that meeting. Each week, the care staff would wheel the resident into the meeting after everyone had arrived and were seated. After several weeks, it was noted by the student observer that the resident being discussed often fell asleep during these team meetings. She observed that except for one brief interchange at the beginning of the meeting when the resident was asked how everything was going and if s/he had any complaints, all further discussion took place among the care team staff. The team realised that, while they had been progressive in recognising the need to include the resident, aside from incorporating his or her physical presence, they had failed to find ways to ensure that this person actually participated in the meeting. One practice identified to redress this was to schedule meetings that would better accommodate the preferences of the resident being discussed. Specifically, they alternated the meeting between mornings one week and afternoons the next – this gave them some flexibility to respond to the time of day that a particular resident was most alert and/or preferred to meet. Additionally, they

established a checklist to be completed by the primary care staff prior
to the meeting to ensure that each resident's unique communication
was understood and responded to in the meeting. Finally active effort
was taken to ensure that all team members were consistently talking
directly to the resident and waiting for his or her response. The team
also began to discuss the possibility of having meetings chaired by
the resident when he or she seemed able and/or interested in taking
on this role.

In this instance it is possible to see how important it is for participation to be not
only maximised but also genuinely valued. A practitioner and/or organisation
must actually want a person to participate and get involved in decisions – doing it
because of a policy or other directive is tokenistic and undermines any attempt to
promote citizenship. However, good intentions alone are not adequate; promoting
and valuing participation also means ensuring adequate resources are in place to
allow a process to unfold that may take longer and be more complicated.

The principle of maximising and valuing participation is not restricted to
personal care decisions. Opportunities are opening up which allow people with
dementia to participate in life in a much broader way, and across a wider spectrum
of forums and issues. Examples of these include membership on service planning
committees, blogging on Alzheimer's society websites, involvement in consultation
events and community advocacy and assisting in training and development of
health and social care professionals. Increasingly, these are the types of activity
that many people with dementia are participating in. Obviously these forms of
participation require different levels of skill, resources and tenacity on the part
of the person with dementia; they also require enlightened practitioners who
have the vision to see and seize potential opportunities for involving those with
dementia and recognising the value of those contributions.

Maximising and valuing participation also recognises that wherever possible
health and social care practitioners avoid speaking on behalf of people with
dementia, but rather strategise to find ways to facilitate so that the voices and
actions of marginalised people themselves are heard and respected. From an anti-
oppressive practice perspective this involves helping an individual: define his/her
own needs; develop the skills and vocabulary required to articulate these needs;
gain access to public forums to address the structures of power base that result in
unmet needs; and to help legitimise these authentic voices by supporting them
in every way possible (Mullaly, 2007, p 302). This is a complicated task when
placed within the context of weakening cognitive abilities and communication
patterns that may no longer function in a conventional manner, as the following
example shows:

When Jenna was diagnosed with dementia in her early 50s, she refused,
as she put it, "to go quietly". Because of her strong advocacy presence
within the community, she was invited to participate on the advisory

board of a local organisation focused on supporting people with dementia. However, she rarely spoke at these meetings and slowly her attendance began to drop off. The chair was concerned about this and spoke to her. It became clear that: (a) she felt quite intimidated as the only non-healthcare professional sitting at the table, especially since she was experiencing word-finding problems related to her dementia; and (b) mornings were a particularly stressful time for her, at least partially because of her medication regime. Based on her input, constitutional changes to the board were implemented that required that there be at least three people with dementia as part of the advisory board (in order to avoid a sense of tokenism and create a stronger climate of peer support). Also, meetings were moved to early afternoon and an escort was arranged to make it easier for Jenna and others volunteering their time to get to the meeting; this required allocating additional funds to the board meetings to ensure the capacity to accommodate.

The objective of maximising the participation of those with dementia is likely to be further complicated by structural issues related to social location. For example, women as a social group have had different experiences than men due to the gendered nature of the labour market. Depending on her stage in the lifecourse, a woman with dementia may never have actively participated in a public meeting or had to speak up for herself before, and may therefore require more (or at least different) assistance than a man with dementia. In addition to this, some older women with dementia may be reluctant to speak out about their care and treatment due to a 'self-perceived lack of education' in relation to professionals who are 'perceived as educated' (Proctor, 2001, p 370). This can, of course, also be the experience for men with dementia. Similarly immigrant or minority ethnic women and men may feel they lack the language skills and/or entitlement to speak out. The point here is that gender, educational background, ethnicity and other social factors such as socioeconomic position across the lifecourse must all be taken into account when the focus is on maximising participation of men and women with dementia. Facilitating active participation for someone whose voice has always been silent (pre-dementia) may be particularly challenging, but also especially worthwhile.

Creating a climate where participation of people with dementia is maximised and valued is a societal responsibility. Some people recognise this (such as those involved in the participatory research project 'Saying Hello', to be discussed later in Chapter Six). However, for others, this will require a fundamental shift in epistemological perspective. Rather than simply trying to find out why any one individual does not participate, it requires a systematic examination of the *conditions* under which the experience of non-participation is produced. This might include, for example, an examination of:

- *Temporal conditions:* how much time is 'allowed' for participation – minutes, hours, days, weeks, months? Do people have the time they need to communicate, particularly in formal meetings and case reviews? Whose time frame is being adhered to when seeking to maximise participation?
- *Spatial conditions:* are people able to move freely in order to participate? How are spaces organised – is there segregation (that is, are there special places for people with dementia)? If so, how does this impact on participation? Are the areas set aside for participation conducive to participation, for example, are they well-designed, well-lit and welcoming places to be? Who determines where people participate?
- *Social conditions:* are people's backgrounds taken into account when promoting participation? How might social statuses impact on a person's propensity to participate?
- *Cultural conditions:* what are the cultural norms around participation? Do particular ways of participation dominate, for example, meetings? Why is that? Are the terms used understandable and meaningful to everyone? Or jargon, embedded in dominant language norms that exclude some? Who determines how people participate and how is that power exercised? What understandings of participation prevail, and do these understandings take account of the embodied knowledge of people with dementia?
- *Policy conditions:* which areas of public policy are relevant to participation? Are these policies implemented? If not, why not? What are the barriers and who are the drivers? To what extent is legislation (such as the NHS Act 2006)[2] used to promote participation?

Organisations that are run by people without dementia (that is, those without a disability) are likely to presume a particular level, and way, of participating in the social world that disadvantages people with dementia. This is because practices and processes will be based on the 'carnal knowledge' of those who are not impaired (rather than those who are) (Paterson and Hughes, 1999). It is only by examining underlying conditions – the conditions that organisational practices are deeply entrenched in – that a climate of participation can be promoted. It cannot be the expectation that people with dementia will adapt to existing conditions; rather, disabling practices and processes must change in order to accommodate people with dementia.

Facilitating growth and creativity in the dementia experience

People with dementia do not stop growing, developing and wanting to experiment just because they are diagnosed with dementia. On the contrary, some people with dementia clearly become more energised and creative as a result of dementia, and this is well demonstrated by people like Rex Marsden, the landscape artist, introduced in Chapter Three, and others like him, such as members of Dementia and Creativity – Light in the Darkness, a group who share photographs on

Flickr. For some people the experience of dementia is a positive one (or at least has positive aspects alongside the negative consequences). This is because, as the following excerpt shows, cognition only ever defines one aspect of the person's experience:

> When Betty describes her experiences with dementia, she discusses her frustration coping with a memory that is no longer dependable. She describes the embarrassment of using inappropriate words or being unable to draw out common, everyday terminology. But she is also quick to note her belief that "It's like the creator takes one thing but gives something else in return" as she discusses the growth in her abilities as an artist and cultural translator. (O'Connor et al, 2009)

A conventional focus on cognition is delimiting. It considers only cranial powers (such as thought, memory, intellect) and forces attention on loss and decline. The personhood literature attempts to soften this focus by stressing how interpersonal environments might facilitate the retention of a sense of self, often by highlighting the importance of 'knowing' the person through their historical preferences, experiences and relationships. However, although promoting a more positive perspective, 'change' is still implicitly perceived in a pejorative way, as something to be feared and avoided. Specifically, the focus, even in the personhood literature, is on 'maintaining' or 'preserving', leaving little room for seeing the dementia experience as a source of growth and development.

A value underpinning a social citizenship approach to practice is that change is lifelong and can continue to occur in positive ways even after a diagnosis of dementia. Individual growth can take many forms, for example spiritual or creative personal development, forming new relationships, improving existing relationships with significant others and/or assuming leadership roles as dementia advocates at broader community and societal levels.

The implications of a more expansive vision on practice that encompasses a focus on growth and development include:

- Practitioners must find ways to create the space to explore growth by recognising diverse personal and cultural interpretations associated with dementia. This would include focused questioning about opportunities for growth and/or change.
- Assessments must be strengths-based rather than deficit-focused. A strengths-based assessment draws attention to those skills and knowledge that are retained and/or have been developed over the lifecourse. These can often provide the springboard for further development.
- Ideal intervention strategies will include exploring opportunities that develop existing skills and knowledge. For example, one important avenue that opens up because of the diagnosis relates to the opportunities available to the person diagnosed to make a difference speaking as a person with dementia. This

has offered an important forum for self-development and growth for some dementia advocates.

- Expressions of hope are re-interpreted and valued. Too often practitioners discourage the maintenance of hope as a sign that the person is not being 'realistic' or 'coming to terms' with their diagnosis. Yet hope allows alternative possibilities to be explored and considered.

Connecting personal experiences to broader sociopolitical and cultural contexts

People's experiences are shaped by broader societal discourses and practices. This means that people's experiences with dementia are not simply responses to the neuropathological changes; they cannot be linearly relegated to personal idiosyncrasies, biographies and/or character traits, nor can they be entirely explained away by problematic interpersonal relationships. Rather, there is growing recognition that individual stories and personal narratives are organised by, and reflect, broader societal discourses and practices: the personal dementia story is no exception.

Attempts to understand and respond to the experiences of people with dementia and their family members must be contextualised within a broader societal level. Interventions are therefore required that focus on change at this level, not just on helping people with dementia and their families to adapt to deterioration related to individual pathology.

> Jack was brought into the geriatric mental health unit for a full assessment at the request of his wife, Glenda. She complained that he was alternating between being increasing belligerent with her, or tearful and withdrawn. Jack sat silently as Glenda discussed her frustration and described a situation the previous day when he had refused to go to church with her. When asked to give his side, he haltingly tried to respond but then began pounding his hand on the sofa as the right words failed to come. With further questioning, Glenda described how uncomfortable their friends had become in Jack's presence, frequently treating him as though he were not there and talking only to her. Even their physician had taken to speaking directly to her, rather than Jack, when discussing Jack's condition and medication needs. She feels uncomfortable with this, but also recognises that the physician is busy and doesn't have the time it would take to talk directly to Jack.

Others have described similar scenarios (see, for example, Sabat, 2001, who discusses this under the label of malignant positioning). In this situation, Jack's increasingly 'disinhibited' behaviour could be described as a symptom of his dementia and treated with medication. In other words, his behaviour might be 'managed'. Unfortunately, as a recent report in the UK shows, this is an all too common response (Banerjee, 2009).

Alternatively, it could be recognised as a societal silencing. When the latter perspective is taken, Jack no longer owns his problem and it no longer makes sense to respond to it as an individual issue. Rather, his 'personal trouble' is seen as reflecting a broader public issue, thereby calling for a response that is multilayered. For example, if Jack's responses are re-interpreted as understandable frustration trying to cope in an ageist and hyper-cognitive society that does not give him time to respond or the benefit of the doubt that he has something to communicate, then at the individual level, Jack needs to know that he is understood and his responses make sense. At the interpersonal level, Glenda requires assistance in finding ways to communicate with Jack that accommodate the deterioration in his verbal skills. She also needs help in identifying appropriate responses for dealing with those situations where the actions of others silence and hurt her husband and leave her feeling angry and uncomfortable. However, while these efforts are important, practitioners need to be careful to move beyond individualising responses. Thus, at a broader level, societal responses and practices that discount the person with dementia by attributing all of their responses to the dementia – even legitimate anger and frustration – need to be challenged. This could be done, for example, by encouraging Glenda to publish a letter in the community newsletter – perhaps anonymously – describing how others' fear and dismissal has hurt her husband. Alternatively, finding ways to make more public those stories and narratives written by others with dementia, who are able to articulate Jack's experience of silencing and disenfranchisement, might facilitate broader social change.

Thus, consistent with the framework presented in Chapter Two, an approach to dementia practice that values social citizenship requires a multidimensional thrust that: (a) recognises that individual problems often reflect broader social issues; and (b) considers subjective (micro) experience, relational (mezzo) environment and sociopolitical (macro) context, and recognises that effective change is required at all three levels.

Often these different layers – particularly the micro/personal and the macro/societal – are considered in isolation. However, when a sociopolitical lens for understanding the dementia experience is applied, the importance of simultaneously working at all levels becomes paramount. At the individual level, this requires making the connection between personal experiences and broader societal practices – or drawing on feminist and disability practice, recognising the personal as political. At the interpersonal level, it requires assisting others to combat societal silencing and stigmatising. This includes developing educational practices that challenge ignorance and fear. At the community level it means changing practices and policies that inadvertently promote destructive understandings and approaches. For example, in the UK, people with dementia and their supporters have fought hard to try and get the government to see that anti-dementia drugs help people to function socially as well as cognitively (see, for example, SDWG,

2007). Finally, at the societal level, it requires challenging language and broader societal practices that marginalise and discount (see Chapter Four).

The implications of this principal for practice include the following:

- Redefining the 'problematics' in direct case-based practice, that is, recognising when individual challenges are symptoms of a broader societal problem. It will still be important to provide case-based support, but this will look different because part of the emphasis will be on normalising responses.
- Determining the level at which intervention can start and then moving iteratively between and among the different levels. This is discussed in further depth later in this chapter.
- Challenging the dichotomy between micro and macro level approaches to practice. In particular, this means finding opportunities at more micro levels of practice to facilitate involvement with change at a broader level.

Promoting solidarity by constructing a 'we' community

Solidarity can be described in terms of a unity of interests between different individuals or groups. Historically, people have tended to unify around the family, work and faith; more recently, however, people are engaging in a greater range and more localised forms of solidarity, as evidenced, for example, by the proliferation of community-based organisations (Thake, 2008). Community-based organisations (such as SDWG and DASNI) are exemplary forms of solidarity, as they grow out of a shared interest (that is, dementia) and seek to bring about social change through individual and collective action.

> I felt disempowered because the people that spoke to me about dementia always spoke about my loss – all the negative things. Nobody ever said "there are things that you've lost but there are also things you could gain". They never really took me from the loss of power into the action. It was the Scottish Dementia Working Group and other people with dementia that did that. I had to find the light at the end of the tunnel. (quoted in SDWG, 2007)

Solidarity is an important aspect of social citizenship: it is all about individuals and groups getting to know each other, sharing strategies and resources, forming coalitions and allegiances, and most importantly, working *together* in order to improve the community in which they live.

The promotion of solidarity and a 'we' community can help people with dementia to feel less alone in their struggle against the disease and associated stigma and discrimination. Further benefits are increased confidence and development of a shared identity (Clare et al, 2008). People depend on others to bolster and endorse alternative ways of understanding and responding, especially when challenging dominant societal norms. Indeed, an approach that focuses generally on building the capacity of a community has many advantages, including:

- *The development of political awareness.* It is easier to link individual issues to broader societal problems when the uniqueness of a person's situation can be questioned and contextualised within a group.
- *Challenging societally imposed identities and stereotypes.* It is easier to contest these, particularly those inherently destructive to a person's sense of self, within a supportive community.
- *Forming and sustaining personally empowering beliefs.* It is easier to form and sustain positive beliefs when those around you are also doing so.
- *Power in numbers.* A group of people can lead the way towards real change in a way that one individual cannot.
- *Re-interpreting problems as shared experiences.* This can result in shifting from needs-based to rights-based expectations for support and services.

Solidarity can be achieved, and strong communities can be built, in many different ways: not everyone with dementia will either want or be able to become a member of an organised group or speak out in public. Rather, a key priority in practice, drawing on ideas of critical social citizenship, is to decrease the isolation that is often such an overarching component of the experiences for people with dementia by facilitating the development of peer networks and coalitions. Unfortunately, in the dementia field, there seem to be limited opportunities to do this. For example, research suggests that family support groups often fail to achieve any empowerment potential because they remain fixated at the level of providing individual support around coping (see, for example, O'Connor, 2002). Similarly, in her study of a support group for people with early dementia, Clare (2002) found little evidence of interaction between members, with most interactions occurring between a member and the (professional) facilitator. Clearly, it is important that people with dementia are empowered and enabled to seek support and strength from each other.

The implications of this principle for practice include the following:

- Where possible, supplement (or replace) individual case-based practice with group-based approaches.
- Conventional group-based approaches need to be challenged to ensure that they are not inadvertently being used to perpetrate an oppressive status quo.
- Thus, while a group format has the potential to move from an individual focus to a more community-based understanding, group leaders require the skills and training to ensure that this potential is realised. Citizenship-oriented practice includes addressing the training needs of group facilitators and leaders to assist them in making the move from mutual support to empowerment.

Towards implementing a critical social citizenship approach to practice

The four principles identified above provide the parameters for developing an approach to dementia practice that is grounded in a critical social citizenship approach. This lens begins with the importance of valuing the person with dementia, but then extends person-centred care practices by explicitly attending to the sociopolitical nature of practice and focusing more explicitly on the agency and status of the person with dementia. We note that these principles are not exclusive to a social citizenship approach – it could be argued that they are equally congruent to a personhood approach. However, as personhood and relationship-based approaches have been conceptualised to date, these ideas are more background, if present at all. Hence, there is a need to explicitly shift focus towards a more sociopolitical perspective that is grounded by anti-oppressive ideas and practices.

In the next section we will broaden the focus from examining how practice *should* look – in other words, articulating principles that in essence, provide practice objectives – to highlighting strategies that have particular promise for ensuring that these principles are achieved. We begin with the premise that some ways of doing practice are more conducive to a social citizenship approach, and it is towards these that we want to draw attention. The remainder of this chapter will focus on three interrelated strategies that we identify as particularly essential for a social citizenship approach to practice. These are: attending to relational power issues; the privileging of narrative approaches; and approaching problem solving using a multidimensional lens. We reiterate that these strategies are not exclusive to a social citizenship approach – aspects of these are discussed, for example, in the person-centred literature. However, in a social citizenship approach, they are all essential and work in tandem.

Strategies for promoting social citizenship:

- Dignifying difference: attending to power in the relationship
- Harnessing the potential of the narrative turn
- Moving towards a multidimensional practice agenda

Dignifying difference: attending to power in the relationship

The foundation for effective dementia practice is the relationship between practitioners, people with dementia and their family or significant others. This is well recognised. Often, however, the power (im)balances within these relationships goes without question. Rather, an implicitly hierarchical power structure is assumed – physicians have the most power, health and social care professionals hold power over the family and the person with dementia and family members hold power over the person with dementia.

In a critical social citizenship approach, attention to the power dynamics within relationships becomes paramount. There are two reasons for this. First, if (as we have argued) an important condition of the dementia experience is the loss of power associated with receiving a diagnosis of cognitive deterioration in a hypercognitive society, then it becomes important from the onset to attend to redressing this situation by creating environments where power is *not* lost. Second, attending to power makes sense: health and social care professionals need to recognise that they are losing important input when they marginalise the voices of people with dementia. Thus, putting into practice the notion that people with dementia can contribute both to their own lives and the well-being of others means, as one husband noted, that professionals need to "take themselves off their pedestals" in order to hear what people with dementia and family members have to say. Within a social citizenship approach to practice, the person with dementia is redefined as a partner and resource rather than simply an individual carrier of problems who must be 'helped'. An authentic and mutually collaborative partnership is the goal.

One step in this process is re-evaluating who is bringing what to the relationship. Historically, in the West, medical wisdom and knowledge has been prioritised over experiential knowledge but a critical social citizenship approach challenges this. Instead, the notion of different but equal knowledge and wisdom becomes important.

Within this context, knowledge can be understood on a continuum from specialised knowledge about some aspects of the general experience – including, for example, medical diagnosis, community service rules and regulations, coping responses and carer stress – to particularised knowledge that is based on a person's own specific situation and experiences. This recognises that a person is the expert of his/her own experiences. The notion of a continuum is used to depict a level and continuous flow of knowledge, implying the importance of all of this knowledge for constructing a holistic and comprehensive understanding. No one set of knowledge is placed above the other. This means that people with dementia and family members – who unquestionably possess the expertise in relation to particularised knowledge – can learn from health and social care practitioners, but it also means that health and social practitioners can learn from people with dementia and their families.

When people with dementia are accorded expertise over the dementia experience, their involvement (on agency boards, for example) becomes less tokenistic, with the recognition that they have something unique and important to offer that the health and social care practitioners do not. Finding ways to hear this input becomes important for all concerned. Thus, the first point here is to recognise the unique knowledge that all partners bring as important and complementary.

A second approach toward equalising relationships is reducing social distance between practitioners and the person with dementia and his/her family. Strategies for doing this include:

- using equitable forms of address, for instance dropping hierarchical titles like referencing some as 'Dr' and everyone else by first names;
- recognising the importance of personal disclosures and being 'real';
- employing direct clear speech that avoids the professional jargon that is so distancing.

Shifting this balance can be challenging depending on the sociocultural background of the person with dementia and his/her family as well as the social location of the practitioner. For example, in some cultures the distance between professionals and the 'patient' is more heavily entrenched, and in many cultures gender socialisations translate into the reality that many feel more intimidated by a male practitioner. On the other hand, practitioners may readily fall into the conventional 'habit' of automatically positioning the person with dementia as a 'client' who needs to be 'helped' – they, too, need to be challenged to look at the dementia diagnosis as the signifier of an unbalanced relationship. This means that addressing social distance between practitioners and people with dementia must be individually negotiated.

A third approach is to provide the knowledge necessary to empower the person with dementia and/or the family members to manoeuvre the system. This could mean providing important information about medical diagnosis and prognosis. It could also mean ensuring that the person is aware of procedures for challenging a decision, has contact information for relevant decision makers such as the local MP and/or advocacy groups and/or is aware of his/her rights in a particular situation. The following example demonstrates how translating knowledge – rather than becoming defensive about practices over which you have no control – can facilitate positive relationships and social change:

> Mr and Mrs Carboni were interested in moving into a shared room at Sunset Manor. Mrs Carboni suffered from dementia and Mr Carboni was finding it increasingly difficult trying to manage her care although he was quite capable of overseeing his own care. However, he was insistent that she was his life; from his perspective they had sworn to be together 'til death did they part' and hence, he felt his only alternative was to go into the facility with his wife. Because their care needs were so different, however, the facility was refusing to consider this. The social worker chose to deal with Mr Carboni's anger first by explaining – but not defending – the rationale behind the facility's decision and then letting him know the procedure for appealing the care team's decision. She assured him that she would not take it personally if he chose to fight the decision. Mr Carboni wrote an eloquent letter to his Member of Parliament and copied it to the head administrator. Unfortunately, he was not able to get the policy changed and his wife was admitted on her own to the care facility. Three years later, however, after several comparable letters, the

administrator reconsidered the policy and delegated two rooms on the heavier care unit to married couples who might have differing care levels. The social worker quietly applauded the action.

A fourth approach for equalising power revolves around consciously attending to and promoting interactions that are more egalitarian. For example, changing risk assessment strategies to incorporate more open-ended structures for obtaining information facilitates more egalitarian interactions in two ways: first, it allows the person with dementia to take some control over what and whose story gets told. Second, a more open-ended structure facilitates better communication by not forcing the person with dementia to conform to conventional responses and ways of communicating. In contrast, standardised approaches to risk assessment limit shared control over the dialogue, allow the practitioner to hear only what s/he wants to hear and prevent important and potentially relevant avenues of communication from opening up. As Roberts (2000, p 433) points out, the 'currently popular outcome measures and risk assessments, plotting individuals on an actuarial scale, are quintessentially modern – rather than postmodern – in the approach and aspirations'. This will be further discussed in the next section examining the merits of using narrative strategically. The point here is to note that how information is obtained during encounters with professionals gives clear messages about who has control.

Health and social care practitioners are placed in a position where they can choose whether or not to take advantage of the power and energy of their so-called 'clients'. When they retain a position of being all-knowing and all-powerful they lose important opportunities, first for facilitating the empowerment of those with whom they are working, and second, for harnessing this energy to facilitate positive change. The 'helping' relationship in which many practitioners encounter people with dementia has historically been hierarchical and practitioners must take action to avoid inadvertently perpetrating relationships that are oppressive, limiting and harmful to people with dementia.

Harnessing the potential of the narrative turn

In Chapter Four we highlighted the power of language for constructing reality and drew attention to how people draw on broader storylines, or discourse, to organise and story their own ways of being in the world. We highlighted the importance of examining the storylines being used to construct our understandings as one means toward challenging taken-for-granted assumptions. We now return to the focus on narrative as an increasingly important strategy for implementing a social citizenship approach to practice. We note that our emphasis on narrative is entirely consistent with innovative work currently under way in the field of dementia studies. Our intention here is to highlight and extend the discussions already beginning around the importance of narrative, by moving beyond the focus on personhood to examine the narrative turn in relation to social citizenship practice. Within this context, narrative can contribute to practice in four ways: as an empowering process; as a means towards essential insights; as an act of community building; and as a focus of change.

First, as discussed in the previous section, a narrative approach to practice can be empowering. For example, narrative assessments clearly position authority and control in the hands of the person telling the story, in this case the person with dementia. This is empowering at the individual level, but also represents an important strategy for subverting the current trend towards increasingly routinised, regimented assessments that can be so dehumanising. For example, in both Canada and the UK the focus on 'evidence-based' practice has too frequently been translated into the use of tools and instruments that lend themselves towards quantifying outcomes. This approach is consistent with the focus on fiscal accountability and cost savings, since structured tools tend to be easier and faster to complete. However, these tools also have an unfortunate tendency to slot people into categories that may not fit and arbitrarily define what is important to know in a particular situation. Thus, narrative as a process can be an effective strategy for maximising participation while simultaneously challenging the sociopolitical status quo.

Second, as has been well developed in the personhood literature, hearing the stories of people with dementia offers essential insight. Practitioners and family members can use this insight to understand the experiences of those with dementia. It may also be useful to others with dementia, including those who are less able to articulate their own stories. As a result of the focus on hearing people's stories over the past 10 years, we have far greater understanding of the issues and experiences of those with dementia.

However, narratives have the potential to offer more than just insight about the individual experience of dementia; they can also offer political insights and opportunities for people to reclaim power and assert authority. To date, there has been a tendency to 'hear' these stories from a more psychological perspective rather than as political statements. Much has been written about the lack of power and control people with dementia have over their lives, but very little about how individuals seek to reclaim it. By speaking out in public, defending and arguing for their rights and commenting on and complaining about care practices, people with dementia are using their voices in a political way to reclaim power and to assert authority. In particular, people are using their voices to reclaim power over an aspect of their lives where they feel they have very little control.

The concept of a political voice is an important one for the field. In some instances it is easy to discern this voice among people with dementia. For example, British people with dementia involved in public campaigns for better care services are clearly using their voices in a political way to reclaim power over their own treatment. However, within specialist care settings, political narratives are perhaps harder to discern. It involves listening, and taking seriously what people have to say about their desires and rights as citizens, that is, as regular members of the community (as opposed to welfare recipient). For example, comments made to

Bartlett (2007) by different people with dementia during her fieldwork in care homes shows what a keen sense some individuals (with quite severe memory problems) have of their status as citizens.

Comment	Citizenship narrative
Once they've got their money, they don't seem to care	Justice
I would like to know more, but I think they think I am an 'old goner'	Discrimination
They'll worry about you; they won't worry about me	Inequality
Do I have to talk to you/tell you about that?	Freedom from obligation
My husband put me in this home. I want a divorce	Loss of control/self-determination
Shall we go out for a drink/walk in the garden?	Freedom to take responsibility

Narratives like these are commonplace in care homes and other specialist care settings; they are significant because they suggest that individuals do have a keen sense of their entitlements and responsibilities as citizens – that is, to be treated fairly and to enjoy certain freedoms. Moreover, they suggest people have an acute sense of fairness and injustice – an important aspect of social citizenship. Unfortunately, comments like these are rarely heard or interpreted in a political way. This is partly because clinical and psychosocial explanations of people's behaviours prevail, particularly in long-term care settings, and partly because sociological concepts are not the frame of reference for most health and social care professionals. Yet, narratives like these must be recognised for what they are, namely, an attempt to reclaim power and control.

In addition to lending insight, a third way that narratives can be used in practice is as a tool for community building. Specifically, narratives facilitate the sharing of insights and perspectives, which brings to light points of similarities with others. Hence, narratives can be used strategically to strengthen collective identity (Davis, 2002, p 19). To some extent, this is already happening within the field of dementia studies at a formal level through organisations such as DASNI. However, there is room for more active efforts by practitioners, through for example, facilitating the development of writing or theatre groups. These have been used within the feminist movement but rarely with people with dementia.

A fourth use for narrative is as the focus of change. To some extent, the use of storying as a means of intervention has a long tradition in gerontological practice, especially in work with people with dementia, through the popularity of reminiscence or life review techniques. However, the focus and use of the story differs between narrative, and reminiscence or life review.

Reminiscence or life review therapy is based on the premise that the recounting and assessment of someone's life is a therapeutic and expectable activity for older people; it is through this retelling that people are able to recognise and validate strengths and life successes, as well as come to terms with the past. With people with dementia, reminiscence is also identified as an important means for helping others to know the person and fostering a sense of continuous self. In contrast, narrative approaches, when grounded by the ideas of post-structuralism, as laid out in Chapter Four, are based on subtly different premises that impact how they can be useful. In particular, life review focuses on the story as a 'true' representation of reality and typically ignores the ways that language and narrative are used as a 'richly complex screen through which perceptions of self and reality are continually filtered' (Ray, 2000, p 26). The difference is that stories understood as objective realities demand passive acceptance, but '(s)tories understood as radically vulnerable can be challenged and re-authored' (Rossiter, 2000, p 27).

This has two implications for practice. First, using this understanding of narrative, the focus in any sort of intervention can move beyond acceptance to actual change. As Ray (2000) notes, since we write ourselves into being, by reinterpreting and rewriting our life stories, we can *change* our way of being. Second, and most importantly to a social citizenship approach, the locus of change shifts from the individual to his/her story and can include a more sociopolitical perspective. Narrative intervention techniques, gaining increasing prominence in the family therapy literature but rarely used in practice with older adults, particularly those with dementia, offer concrete techniques that can facilitate the shift from individualising an issue to moving it outside of a person's self to a broader sociopolitical landscape. Externalising is one such process. Here, through careful focus on language use and reframing, a problem is objectified and given a name, or personified so that it can then be talked about as though an objective entity outside of the person. The goal is to separate the person from the problem in such a way as to make the problem the problem rather than the identity of the person the problem (White and Epston, 1990).

One way to do this is to take advantage of the biomedical discourse to medicalise the problem:

> Mrs Cook spoke quietly of the shame she felt that her husband no longer recognised her. She felt that this lack of recognition must speak to the quality of her relationship with her husband. Surely if she had been a better wife he would not have forgotten who she was! Identifying the problem as an example of 'the dementia' at work challenged this perception. She was able to begin to depersonalise the symptoms as somehow reflective of her own inadequacy and instead, began to look for ways that she could minimise the power of the invading dementia.

As this example demonstrates, using the 'dementia' label selectively can be useful. However, it can also be risky because this understanding is already so powerful that it can take over the person – as already demonstrated. The challenge associated with externalising is to use the process as a means for constructing a new understanding that is empowering. Ways towards achieving this include mapping the influence that the person has had on the problem and not just focusing on the power the problem has over the person. The intent is to reconstruct damaging stories about a person by drawing on other perhaps more hidden ways of understanding and interpreting. For example:

> Jack Brooks is an 82-year-old, retired professor who lives alone. After living in fear for the past several years that he was "losing it", he was ultimately diagnosed with dementia eight months ago. Since then he has become increasingly despondent, including giving up writing, an activity that he previously spent at least four hours per day working on. At the request of his daughter, a community health nurse visited him in his home. Dr Brooks described feeling like he was "going crazy" and that slowly he was "losing himself"; he questioned that he would be better off dead. The community nurse focused first on helping him to externalise the issue to recognise that 'he' was not going crazy, rather dementia was 'invading' his brain. A series of mapping questions were then asked in order to examine alternative ways of understanding the situation: "How has dementia convinced you of your helplessness? How did you beat dementia enough to speak out today? What would help you to combat the influences of the dementia?" Through this process, Dr Brooks began to see that part of the problem was related to how others were treating him as though he had nothing further to say. He shifted his focus in writing to begin to document his experiences.

Other strategies for fostering this restorying are well developed in the narrative therapy literature and could usefully be integrated into practice with people with dementia and their families.

However, there are particular challenges in applying a narrative approach in practice with people with dementia. Specifically, these approaches as they have been defined to date typically focus on the spoken language. This represents an area where people with dementia may experience considerable difficulty. Communication problems such as word-finding, difficulty in representing more abstract thinking and distractibility are just some of the issues that routinely interfere with the communication attempts of people with dementia. Historically, there has been some tendency to dismiss what people with dementia are saying as a result of these difficulties. Trying to listen beyond words to capture the meaning of the speaker can be hard work. It becomes easy to assume that because the person cannot communicate in a conventional manner that s/he has little to communicate.

It is obviously important to recognise that people with dementia do have something important to say, and there is a growing body of literature focused on helping people to say what they want to say (see, for example, Killick and Allan,

2001). In addition to these, Baldwin (2008) proposes three ways that we might move beyond communication problems to consider narrative citizenship in a way that fosters the narrative agency of people living with dementia in the 'narrative enterprise'. The first is to seek other symbolic means of expression – to move beyond spoken language to consider for example, the importance of embodied communication; that is, to recognise that people speak themselves through their bodily movements and actions, not just through words. As Baldwin (2008, p 225) notes, 'stories can be articulated as much through dance movement and artistic expression as they can language – if we as readers are sensitive enough to the narrative features of such media'. Second, practitioners can look towards joint authorship where narrative processes are shared or co-constructed (Williams and Keady, 2006) and a final narrative is 'a deliberate and consciously negotiated product between those people living with dementia and others, or a piecing together of the fragmented narratives of the person living with dementia by those who support them' (Baldwin, 2008, p 225). The third way is to: '… see the here and the now impact of the person with dementia on the emerging stories of those around them'. For example, some carers report that following the onset and progression of dementia for their relative, they (the carers) become more patient, tolerant and so on. Thus, the person with dementia contributes to the story of another (Baldwin, personal communication). Combined, these approaches highlight the importance of finding ways to recognise narrative agency among people with dementia that moves beyond spoken language.

At first glance, the previous focus on personal narrative might seem to support a focus on individual subjectivity rather than a critical social analysis necessary for anti-oppressive practice. However, returning to the notion of discourse as discussed in Chapter Four, a post-structural understanding of narrative suggests that personal stories do not simply reflect individual experiences; they are organised according to culturally available, but tacit 'reasoning procedures' (Widdicombe, 1993). This means that the personal story reflects the beliefs, ideas and messages to which someone has been exposed as they have interacted with their familiar, social, political, economic, spiritual and cultural milieus. Drawing on Foucault's (1980) notion of practices of power, they expose the 'grand narratives' that are operating and challenge the authority of those grand narratives (White and Epston, 1990).

Listening with a critical ear to personal narratives, then, not only makes visible the individual's experience but also helps to contextualise that experience within a broader sociopolitical context. This understanding has enormous implications for a critical social citizenship practice in the field of dementia studies. As Baldwin (2008, p 224) highlights, linking narrative to a wider sociology can account for both the narrative construction of personhood and the citizenship issues of power, social inclusion and agency. Thus, while at one level externalising can be limited to exposing the person's relationship with the issue and finding new ways to understand and move forward, at another level, second order externalising focuses on unmasking the societal issues that defined and maintain the client problem systems. This moves away from a focus on an individual with a problem into the role of 'group member constrained by social forces' (Vodde and Gallant, 2002, p 445). Hence, employing narrative strategies in individual casework has the potential to begin the process of politicising an issue and creating a stronger sense of a 'we' community.

In summary, privileging narrative approaches is especially congruent for realising a social citizenship approach for a number of reasons. As a *process*, they facilitate a more egalitarian relationship between people with dementia and others, including health and social care practitioners; in terms of *content*, they provide the knowledge necessary to really 'hear' what people with dementia have to say on two levels – the personal and the sociocultural; as a practice *intervention*, they suggest ways for developing case-based practice that avoid the trap of individualising issues while still recognising the need for individualised responses; and as an *outcome*, if used strategically, they can facilitate political voice and solidarity among people with dementia.

Combined, a major advantage of narrative approaches is that they offer a viable means for challenging the individual/social dichotomy that has so frequently characterised health and social care practice. The individual is seen both as a product but also a co-constructor of social reality. It no longer makes sense to isolate personal change from broader societal change. Rather, the two become intertwined. This then leads to the third strategy for implementing the principles of a social citizenship approach to practice: finding ways to do practice that simultaneously facilitate attention to individual needs and social change.

Moving towards a multidimensional practice agenda

A critical social citizenship approach to practice requires explicitly linking personal problems related to the experience of dementia to broader sociopolitical issues. This requires that social and health care practitioners adapt a lens for practice that is flexible and multidimensional, recognising that intervention may be required, and is possible, on a variety of levels. Under the umbrella of empowerment-oriented practice, Cox and Parsons (1994) describe one such approach for working with older adults:

> Empowerment-oriented practice may be conceptualized on a continuum of focus that ranges over the personal, interpersonal, environment and political aspects of the problem at hand. Focus on the problem may fluctuate from personal to political and from political to personal; however, all dimensions are critical to the empowerment process. The goal of empowerment-oriented practice is the most comprehensive analysis and approach possible for each problem-solving situation. (p 50)

Their four-dimensional approach – individual, interpersonal, environmental and political – can be readily adapted to the dynamic, multidimensional model proposed in Chapter Two that considered subjective experience (individual), interactional environment (interpersonal relationship and immediate physical environment) and sociocultural context (broader social environment, structures and discourses).

Table 5.1 adapts and develops the ideas originally proposed in Cox and Parsons' (1994) empowerment model in order to frame a multidimensional social citizenship approach to dementia practice.

The purpose of this table is to provide ideas about how a multidimensional level of practice might look. The dimensions do not progress linearly; rather, the practitioner may become involved at any level, depending on the situation. This is important because it provides a lens for explicitly seeing people with dementia as something other than clients or people in need. It opens up the space for practitioners to have different types of relationships. Two examples are used to illustrate this:

> Mrs Shemani, a 68-year-old Iranian immigrant, lives alone in a small basement apartment in a high crime area of the city. A referral was made to the mental health team by the physician based on concerns that Mrs Shemani, diagnosed with dementia two years ago, was becoming isolated and seemed to be having increasing difficulty managing at home. A community worker visited her in her home and encouraged her to 'tell her story' – the worker discovered a still articulate woman who had been a teacher in Iran before being forced to seek asylum in Canada. Since immigrating some 20 years earlier, she had been restricted to working in a low-paying domestic position because of language proficiency requirements, and was now living well below the official poverty line since her retirement. Her sponsor, a widowed daughter, had recently been diagnosed with cancer and was in no position to assist financially or emotionally. The worker chose not to focus on the dementia as the main issue. Instead, she: (a) helped Mrs Shemani manoeuvre the government bureaucracy required to seek increased financial subsidy; and (b) connected Mrs Shemani to a recently formed older women's immigrant group who were attempting to increase cultural sensitivity and knowledge within the local community – this included advocating on Mrs Shemani's behalf for travel subsidy through a local Immigrant Society, recognising that it was unsafe for her to try to get to the meetings without support. The worker acknowledged that Mrs Shemani had important and unique insights to offer both as an older immigrant woman and as someone experiencing dementia. She also hoped that Mrs Shemani might connect with two other women in the early stages of dementia who currently attended this meeting. Later, the worker sought out this group, including Mrs Shemani, as an important resource to help her develop an educational pamphlet about dementia that could be translated in Farsi.

Table 5.1: A multidimensional approach to 'intervention'

Dimension of focus	Bridging task	Problem-solving activities	Primary target for change	Primary role of practitioner
Individual (subjective experience)	Examine link between individual areas of difficulty and: a) immediate interactional environment; b) broader sociopolitical context	Relationship-building Assess needs Address immediate discomforts Begin process of reframing issues and consciousness-raising	Individual experiences and perceptions	Support and assistance to person with dementia and his/her family members
Interpersonal relationships	Examine how relationships are being supported/constrained by: a) resource allocation b) sociocultural discourses c) each partner's issues/needs	Knowledge and skills development Connecting and community building (group work)	Interpersonal relationships	Leader, facilitator and educator
Community	Examine how an individual with dementia is being supported/constrained by: a) physical environment b) opportunities for meaningful involvement c) community practices and policies Examine how community practices are organised by broader social discourses	Foster and support involvement of people with dementia in decision-making capacities and leadership roles Reveal oppressive policies and practices and their impact	Environment Organisational policies and practices	Advocate Community development Social change agent
Sociopolitical	Examine impact of broader policies and practices on lived experiences (case-specific and general) Analyse texts (including media) as individual structuring practices	Identify and assist in removing structural barriers which prevent full participation Work with networks and grass-roots organisations Articulate political nature of personal problems Promote collective action (including encouraging letter writing; involving media…)	Societal discourse	Advocate Social change agent Consultant

Source: Adapted from a table initially proposed by Cox and Parsons (1994, p 52) entitled 'Four-dimensional conceptualisation of focus of intervention'.

This first example begins at the individual level, and adapts a more conventional approach to practice. In this example, helping Mrs Shemani is the focus. In contrast, this second example takes a different start point. It recognises how people can indirectly benefit from approaches that are broader in focus:

> Sunset Villa, a nursing home catering to people in more advanced stages of dementia, was committed to developing a facility that was truly person-centred. In order to assist in the educational process, the facility decided to create a teaching video identifying ways of communicating that were more person-centred. The video would feature a resident living in the facility. Of all the residents, John O'Hara, a somewhat disengaged, wheelchair-bound, 91-year-old man in the advanced stages of dementia, was identified as someone who might enjoy the experience; he could not give informed consent but his son readily agreed. A video was produced – part of which involved using Mr O'Hara's personal narrative, including pictures, to demonstrate the importance of understanding a person from a lifecourse perspective, as a continuous and evolving person. For the next few years the video was shown to existing staff and used as a training tool for inter-professional students. Mr O'Hara's status on the unit changed as he became somewhat of a celebrity. Moreover, staff felt more connected to him because they had both a better understanding of who he was, as well as a repertoire of knowledge to facilitate access to his inner world. One result of this experience was that the need for practices and policies to be implemented that helped create a full portrait of each resident living at Sunset Manor was recognised as a priority.

So exploring and understanding the issues using a multidimensional framework offers potentially novel ways of responding. While the person with dementia may individually feel the discomfort, the cause and best response cannot be assumed to be best situated at the individual level. A multidimensional lens allows practitioners to work more creatively, and less pejoratively, with people with dementia and their situations.

Conclusion

Using a social citizenship lens for understanding dementia directs attention to power and disempowerment. If power, or loss of power, is a central feature of the dementia experience then practice in the field of dementia must take anti-oppressive, empowerment-oriented approaches. Empowerment-oriented practice engages people with dementia in actions that challenge or change the personal, interpersonal and political aspects of their life situation. In broadening the debate around dementia practice, the importance of including an explicitly sociopolitical perspective becomes paramount. In this chapter we have outlined some key principles and strategies for working and intervening in this kind of way.

Note

[1] The term 'critical' social and health care practices is being used to reference those approaches that include an explicitly anti-oppressive lens which links personal experiences to the broader sociopolitical and cultural context. These approaches go by different names but include approaches such as feminist practice, structural social work and anti-oppressive practice.

[2] The NHS Act 2006 places a statutory duty on NHS organisations to consult with patients when planning or considering the reorganisation of services.

Extending research practices

Introduction

There is growing emphasis on developing practices and understandings that are informed by research. Often this is discussed under the guise of 'evidence-based' practice, but it is also reflected in discussion about ensuring that research is designed, conducted and disseminated in such a way that it is relevant to those for whom it is intended. The focus of this chapter is on examining the implications and applications of a social citizenship lens for research practices in the area of dementia studies. It is not about how to achieve evidence-based practice, or how to do social research per se, although conventional aspects of this work, such as locating evidence, methods of data collection and analysis, are discussed. Rather, the intent is to highlight how research-related practices might be recast and extended in order to integrate a social citizenship lens. In particular, the chapter examines the ways in which some of the components of citizenship outlined in Chapter Three, namely, meaningful participation and freedom from discrimination, might be located or realised in the different phases of designing, conducting and/ or using social research.

Consistent with the overall theme of this book, this chapter argues for a broader, more ambitious vision in relation to the process of locating, designing, conducting, disseminating and using social research. We begin with the premise that we must 'EXPECT' that men and women with dementia can, and should, be actively involved with the generation and translation of new knowledge. However, to realise this expectation requires that we (re)consider what we regard as evidence, what we research, how we research and where we take the knowledge that is generated through research. The remainder of this chapter will address these questions of what, how, where and by whom, using the heuristic framework EXPECT, for (re)considering the essential elements of the research process in a way that brings a social citizenship lens to the fore.

EXPECT framework for locating social citizenship in research:

- **E**vidence-based practice reconsidered: privileging people's stories
- e**X**tended research agenda
- **P**articipatory and creative methods
- **E**thical debates and dilemmas
- **C**ritical lens
- **T**ranslation of research into practice

E: Evidence-based practice reconsidered

One way in which the notion of citizenship can be located in research is to reconsider the value of evidence derived from people with dementia and their family members. Historically, in debates about evidence-based practice, evidence derived from systematic reviews of randomised controlled trials (RCTs) has been regarded as the 'best' source of evidence. Many standard texts on the topic include a 'hierarchy of evidence' that has experiments or random controlled studies at the top and evidence derived from other sources, such as personal experience, at the bottom. Evidence derived from RCTs is revered because methodologically it is seen as the gold standard for adhering to traditional positivistic standards such as reducing bias and promoting generalisability of findings, and because philosophically it fits with a biomedical approach to health, where the notion of evidence-based practice originated (Hamer and Collinson, 2005). However, in recent years, the idea of a 'hierarchy of evidence' has been critiqued and in some cases replaced with the notion of a continuum of evidence, with quantitative approaches at one end and qualitative at the other.

In thinking about a continuum of evidence it is important to differentiate between knowledge based on professional expertise and that derived from personal experiences (of living with dementia). Both sources of evidence are important, although professional expertise has historically carried more weight. However, in recent years the status of evidence derived from personal stories has risen quite dramatically, as government agencies and professional bodies strive to collect and make available subjective accounts of illness. Some of these are outlined below in Figure 6.1.

Figure 6.1: A selection of online databases of personal stories

- NHS Choices is a UK government website. It contains people's experiences of living well with different health conditions. The site includes Peter van Spyk's story of being diagnosed with dementia: www.nhs.uk/livewell/dementia/pages/dementiarealstory.aspx
- Healthtalkonline is a UK-based charity that collects and makes available online individuals' personal experiences of health and illness. The site includes the experiences of family carers of people with dementia: www.healthtalkonline.org
- A Royal College of Nursing project entitled 'Patient Voices', which seeks to place patients' stories at the heart of healthcare. Dementia-related stories include 'From darkness into light: new worlds': www.pilgrim.myzen.co.uk/patientvoices/find.htm

Online databases like these demonstrate not only the increasing importance given to personal stories in relation to research information, but also that when men and women with dementia do voice their experiences, the impact can be quite powerful – more powerful, and memorable, perhaps, than the reading of a scientific paper.

Unfortunately, however, while there have been great strides towards a research agenda that incorporates the voices of men and women with dementia as personal experts, there is still some distance to go to ensure that the type of 'evidence' derived through this process carries the same weight as other types of research-based knowledge. This is partly because the privileging of knowledge derived from professional/disciplinary experience continues to run very deep in practice, and partly because evidence derived from people with dementia can still be dismissed on grounds that it is, for example, 'too subjective', derived from sample sizes that are too small for 'generalisability', and that it fails to control for extraneous variables. In other words, traditional positivistic standards continue to prevail, even though personal stories are increasingly seen as important.

As one step towards achieving research practices that are more congruent with a social citizenship lens, this privileging of methods that limit or discount the power of the voices of people with dementia must be challenged. Some next steps could include:

1) The development of community research advisory boards to examine how funding structures – particularly those committed to promoting the rights of people with dementia (that is, Alzheimer's societies) – may inadvertently continue to prioritise some approaches to research over others in a way that is pejorative to valuing the input of people with dementia. This could include for examining how language and/or formatting is used to ensure that knowledge based on personal experiences is valued. It is often clear by looking at the structure of the application framework or proposal guidelines that a funding body is privileging a positivist paradigm – for example, research participants are referred to as 'subjects', there is an emphasis on identifying how 'controls' will be used, and the proposal calls for a hypothesis.

2) Recognising that policy makers do value numbers, and so encourage research that begins to pull together the many narratives that now exist through, for example, secondary meta-analysis of qualitative exploratory studies. Worldwide there is a huge database derived from small studies that would carry much more weight if there were ways of integrating it. This would, of course, require that researchers show leadership and collaborate internationally.

X: eXtended research agenda

To date the scope of most social research in the dementia field has been directed at transforming the quality of health and social care. Even in debates about making research practices more inclusive, the assumption has been that improved quality care will be the goal. On the one hand, a focus on care-related issues by researchers is understandable, as there is so much to do in terms of health and social service development. On the other hand, however, focusing only on care issues prevents a move towards a broader vision and understanding of people's *lives*. For example, while the focus is on care, little knowledge is being generated about how differently dementia affects a person's lifestyle, such as their role at work and within their social networks and community. To ensure that people's broader experiences as general citizens are properly recognised and understood the field must extend the research agenda by expanding the range of topics and issues that are being addressed.

Arguing for an extension to the research agenda is consistent with wider policy directives and academic debates. For instance, the UN *Research agenda on aging for the 21st century* identifies 'care systems' as just one of the critical research arenas – it identifies nine others, including: social participation and integration; economic security; macro-societal change and development; healthy ageing; quality of life; changing structures and functions of families, kin and community; and policy process and evaluation (UN Programme on Ageing and the International Association of Gerontology, 2007). In addition, disability scholars have long been calling for a research agenda that encompasses societal issues, such as discrimination, rather than just individual experiences of care. Underpinning these calls is an awareness that (older) people with a disability are at risk of being homogenised by research practices if wider issues are not taken into account. Thus, extending the research agenda is one way of elevating the status of people with dementia.

Taking into account the topics proposed by the UN in relation to a general ageing agenda, as well as what is already known about work under way in dementia research and disability studies, three areas are identified as particularly salient directions for dementia research to take using a social citizenship lens: understanding and combating stigma and discrimination related to cognitive deterioration; understanding and addressing topics related to work – paid and unpaid; and exploring transportation and travel issues.

Stigma and discrimination associated with cognitive impairments

As mentioned earlier in this book, people with dementia are entitled to experience freedom from stigma and discrimination, and some individuals probably do. Unfortunately, despite high-quality work over the past two decades, societal attitudes towards people with dementia remain extremely stigmatising and discriminatory. Those affected by dementia are still often seen as 'tragic', weak and completely incapable, and the popular media, in particular, continues to represent 'dementia' as a catastrophe and death sentence. This does not help the millions of people who are living with dementia across the world to move forward.

Empirical studies find that many people with dementia feel stigmatised and are aware of negative ideas held about them (Barnett, 2000; Gillies, 2000; Pratt, 2002; Hulko, 2005; Bartlett, 2007; Langdon et al, 2007). Younger people with dementia face the additional attitudinal barrier of disbelief, as dementia is still regarded as an 'old person's disease', even by medical and allied health professionals (Alzheimer's Society, 2008). People with dementia from non-Western cultures, and those who have experienced social inequalities such as poverty all their life, may face additional disadvantage.

Research is emerging that is beginning to illuminate how people cope in the light of a disabling condition; this is useful and important. However, finding out how people 'cope with' disabling attitudes is not the only issue. A research priority must also include identifying and eradicating the disabling attitudes that men and women with dementia still have to face. In this research agenda, society – and its injurious attitudes, beliefs and practices – becomes the subject of the research. For example, we know we live in a 'hyper cognitive society' (Post, 2000) but how can pejorative societal attitudes linked to 'hyper cognition' be uprooted and changed? What are the social processes and attitudes that serve to *dis*able those living with dementia from reaching their full potential and remaining actively engaged across the life span? In addition, research suggests that dementia is feared (Corner and Bond, 2004), but what exactly is the basis of that fear, what anxieties do the public have about dementia, and how do these fears limit people with dementia? Moreover, what can be done to allay people's fears and anxieties?

Work: paid and unpaid

Work, whether it is paid or unpaid, is arguably the single most important aspect of being a citizen. Having a job is a source of positive identity, status and stability and can help people with a disability feel a valued part of society (Roulstone and Barnes, 2005). For many, employment – paid and unpaid – gives meaning and structure to their life. Moreover, in addition to its intrinsic value for the sense of self, there are economic advantages to having regular employment that impact on every aspect of a person's life experiences and opportunities. Yet, despite the significance of this topic, this sphere of life remains somewhat of a mystery in the dementia field. The impact of dementia on working life and people's ability to contribute economically and practically to society is rarely discussed. When work life is discussed, it is generally only within the context of younger people with dementia; the productivity of older adults is rarely considered.

This lack of attention is partially because it is assumed that this issue has little relevance to people with dementia. Wider public discourse has assumed that people with dementia do not work or volunteer – either because they are too old and/ or cognitively impaired, or because the labour market has no real opportunities suitable for someone with dementia. This prejudice can be seen, for example, when examining the formula used to calculate the economic burden to society related to dementia often used in research; here, a spouse's or other family member's lost income is included in the model but not the lost income of the person with dementia. The reality is that a sizeable proportion of the population with dementia is likely still to be employed when they first experience the signs of, and are subsequently diagnosed with, dementia. Further, those aged over 65 may still be working, either in a paid or voluntary capacity, and indeed, employment and volunteering opportunities may well have increased and intensified for some *because they have a diagnosis of dementia* – think how incredibly busy some people with dementia are in campaigning, educational and other work-related activities. Clearly it is important that research broadens to investigate the sphere of employment and volunteering.

Limited research has begun to explore this. One useful source of evidence is a UK-based report entitled *Out of the shadows* (Alzheimer's Society, 2008). In this report a number of individuals talk candidly about the effects of dementia on their working life. For example, one person described the impact of diminishing cognitive function on his ability to teach: 'I was struggling at work.... I was losing track and losing control of the class which is something I had never done. I became disorganised, which again is something I have never done' (p 17). This research suggests that issues related to work – both paid and voluntary – do impact on the experience of dementia. From both a social citizenship and lifecourse perspective, it would be useful to know more about the significance of these events on people's experiences of dementia and to ask questions such as: how is 'retirement' different when it is precipitated by a dementia? How does 'work' continue after leaving the realm of paid employment? What structural modifications are required in order to facilitate access of people with dementia to both the paid and unpaid workforce? How effectively is employment and disability or human rights legislation being applied to protect the rights of people with dementia?

Of particular concern is the link between employment and socioeconomic impact. There are clear links already established regarding the influence of socioeconomic factors on health and well-being within the mainstream ageing literature, but little research has investigated this link specifically in relation to dementia. It would be useful, for instance, if there were a programme of research on the socioeconomic impact of developing dementia, as evidence about this is patchy. One study found that people could soon find themselves in financial hardship if they did not seek and obtain a diagnosis (see Walton, 1999). But it is not clear how current or widespread this experience is or whether those on a low income face particular issues or problems when diagnosed with dementia.

Travel and transport

Being able to travel and access transport services is an integral part of being a free citizen. Travel and public transport is a particularly important issue for people with dementia, as many have to stop driving because they begin to find it stressful or they lose confidence and/or competence (UK Alzheimer's Society factsheet 439). Empirical work indicates a link between travel and transport for social citizenship, as one of the few studies on this topic, conducted in the US, found that no longer being able to drive leads to a diminishment of social participation and sense of loss for most people (Taylor and Tripodes, 2001). From a disability perspective, the problem that needs to be addressed here is not how someone with a cognitive impairment copes with not being able to drive but how society must start to address the transport needs of a growing subsection of society.

Lack of accessible public transport is seen as a barrier to people with a disability participating actively in their local communities and accessing local amenities and services. Similarly, in the dementia field, lack of public transportation is cited as a particular issue for people with dementia and their families living in rural areas (Wenger et al, 2002); the Social Exclusion Unit (2006) suggests that better public transport and local taxi vouchers could help ensure that people with dementia are able to get out and about within their local neighbourhood (p 94). However, while these reports make clear the importance of accessible transportation to quality of life, participation and well-being, what 'accessible' transportation looks like in the face of cognitive loss remains unclear. For example, how accessible is public transportation to someone who may no longer be able to manage bus schedules and/or find their way home from bus stops? How do people with dementia get around after a driving licence is revoked? How might bus schedules and information be modified in order to accommodate changes in cognitive and visual functioning related to dementia (as well as those related to ageing)?

Summary

Stigma, work-related issues and travel and transport issues are but three potential topics for further research. People with dementia are a growing subset of society facing an increasingly wide range of challenges and successes. It is imperative that researchers think 'outside the box' when designing research projects and programmes of work. This is particularly important now, as issues related to dementia seem to be very much on the agenda (see, for example, the Nuffield Council on Bioethics, 2009). However, a disproportionate amount of funding continues to be directed toward the three Cs – cause, cure and care. While this is important, so are other aspects of life.

P: Participatory and creative methods

The shift towards personhood has resulted in more importance being placed on including people with dementia in the research process. It is no longer acceptable to presume that a person cannot participate in a research study or service evaluation simply because they have a dementia diagnosis. On the contrary, there is a growing commitment, both in the dementia community and beyond, to involve people with dementia in every aspect of the research and evaluation process to the fullest extent possible. This is evidenced in the UK, for instance, by the Quality Research in Community Network, a collective group of 170 people with dementia and family care partners set up by the Alzheimer's Society, whose role is to comment on research applications and processes, to help set the organisation's research priorities and to monitor ongoing projects funded by the organisation. Similarly, the Dementias and Neurodegenerative Diseases Research Network (DeNDRoN) is keen to involve 'patients, carers and others in its research activities' (for further details see INVOLVE at www.invo.org.uk/). The research community is clearly trying to find ways to endorse and promote the participation of people with dementia in research-related activities.

However, despite current activities and best intentions there is still much more work to do on the research practice front to ensure that research practices are – drawing on a guiding research directive used by the person-centred Murray Alzheimer Research and Education Program (MAREP) – conducted both *for* and *by* people with dementia. For instance, there are surprisingly few opportunities for people with dementia to actually determine for themselves the nature of their engagement in a research or service evaluation project. Often a person with dementia comes on board in research projects only after the research questions and methods have already been developed, and their role becomes that of a 'subject' expected to complete a standardised form, and/or be interviewed or observed in the way the researcher sees fit. Such practices are treating people with dementia as 'passive research subjects' (as opposed to active social agents) and may further marginalise them rather than promote their participation.

Of course, it is not just the way in which research is conducted that can be an issue. Context can also challenge a focus on participant involvement. For example, researchers are often under so much pressure by funders, their own institutions, ethics committee and other powerful bodies to conduct research in a particular way, and within certain time frames, that participants (with any kind of disability) can end up feeling alienated and oppressed by the whole process.

One way of ensuring research practices chime with the principles of social citizenship is to take a participatory approach. Participatory research can be described as an approach to knowledge generation that responds to the importance of doing research *with* and *for* participants rather than on them: it sees the 'active involvement of participants as beneficial and necessary' and encourages active involvement in all aspects of the process, from research design to dissemination (Silver, 2008, pp 102/105). A good example of this approach involving older people is the 'Saying Hello' project in Wigan, England: volunteer researchers (older people themselves) were recruited by a local university and Age Concern, trained, and then, in partnership with the researchers, developed a research programme about avoiding isolation and loneliness.[1]

A participatory approach to research is concerned first and foremost with *how* the research is conducted, rather than which particular methods are used to collect data (Henderson, 1995, p 61; emphasis added). It is concerned with 'how' because of the risks inherent in taking an uncritical approach to research – namely, oppression, disempowerment, silencing and so forth. Above all, a participatory approach to research is concerned with the 'political aspects' of knowledge production (Reason, 1994). Hence, this approach to research is a particularly good fit with social citizenship values and goals.

Much has been written about participatory research, particularly in the fields of disability studies, where historically research participants have been unable to participate fully or meaningfully due to the dominant, oppressive research practices of non-disabled researchers (see, for example, Stone and Priestley, 1996). At its furthest extreme, this has included querying the involvement of non-disabled researchers in disability research. More moderate approaches have raised awareness of how conventional research strategies can silence people with disability, often quite unintentionally. For example, Booth and Booth (1996, p 63) highlight the potential for an interview to become more like 'an interrogation' for participants with learning difficulties, as some researchers find it hard to value or cope with long silences. The same danger arguably exists in interview-based studies involving people with dementia. The issue among scholars who argue for a participatory approach is that people with disabilities lack ownership over the production of knowledge, even though the knowledge produced is about them. Moreover they see power and control in the hands of researchers, when it should be with those who are being researched.

Addressing the massive imbalance of power that often exists between researcher and participant, particularly those who have any kind of disability or mental health condition, lies at the heart of a participatory approach to research (Trivedi and Wykes, 2002). The goal for participatory researchers must therefore be to ensure that the relationships they have with participants are equal ones. This can be achieved in a number of ways. For example, people with dementia who have been involved in research studies have gone on to write about their experiences, thereby becoming an equal voice within the research community (see, for example, Robinson, 2002; McKillop and Wilkinson, 2004). Or equality might be achieved through reciprocal acts: one of the authors (RB) is currently taking photographs of people with dementia involved in campaign activities as part of her fieldwork; she prints some of the images she has taken and gives a copy to participants. Of course, levels of participation in participatory research will always vary. They might vary due to the effects of dementia, or due to the busy lifestyles that people lead.

Participatory research demands that attention to power and participation ground the entire research process: from beginning to target what will be researched, to how it will be researched and finally, to how it will be used. Moore et al (1998) propose the following critical thinking points and questions to assist those undertaking participatory research in working through this process (see Figure 6.2).

Developing the potential of participatory approaches within the field of dementia represents an exciting but formidable challenge. The field of participatory research is itself still developing. Opportunities and strategies for adapting the process in order to respectfully accommodate cognitive changes related to dementia brings special challenges. For example, not uncommonly, a project will take several years from start to finish: how can these time realities be meshed with a deteriorating condition? Are there ways of structuring involvement to ensure an ebb and flow of individual involvement while maintaining coherence to that involvement? How can often competing language requirements be approached? For example, a sort of 'research speak' is often required to convince funding bodies that the research team possesses the necessary skills and knowledge to carry out a project. This is not the same language non-researchers speak, and may pose a particular problem when a person is already coping with communication challenges related to dementia. How can research teams adjust? How can funding bodies modify their expectations to accommodate these differences? These represent only some of the

Figure 6.2: Reflexive questions to set in motion a participatory approach to research

General

- How do you create alliances with people with dementia and how do people with dementia create alliances with you?[a]
- How can you place your methodological expertise in the hands of those who may wish to use research to combat stigma and discrimination?[a]
- Who do you feel accountable to – people with dementia, your employer, funder?
- Who has power over your research activities?[a]
- What are the interests of those who have such power?[a]
- If power relations are oppressive, who are your allies, and who can help you to resist undesirable levels of control over your work?[a]
- List some of the rights you consider essential for people with dementia in a research project. Think about why you have selected these[a]
- What mechanisms can be put into place to ensure these rights are safeguarded in your research project?[a]

Pre-data collection

- Why do you want to collect data in the way you are proposing?
- How can you involve people with dementia in the design of your research?
- If someone with dementia asks you what the research is for, how will you respond?
- What assumptions do you make when designing your research – for example, that people won't be able to give consent or use technologies?

During data collection

- How might you modify procedures and techniques to enable participation?
- What strategies can be used to ensure that people with dementia do not experience alienation from the research process?

Post-data collection

- What can you do to ensure people with dementia are involved in the dissemination of findings?
- What has changed for people with dementia as a result of your research?
- Will there be opportunities for people with dementia to critique your research?

Source: [a] Questions adapted from Moore et al (1998)

questions that remain largely unanswered within the field. Participatory research is clearly an ideal, but we have a long way to go to ensure that it becomes a reality. One place where ideals associated with participatory research methods seems to be making faster inroads is in developing the potential of data collection tools to address power issues. The focus here is on expanding the repertoire of data generation strategies. Expanding the way we do research will help to maximise participation and thereby promote a sense of citizenship.

A first step towards this has been to explore the potential of in-depth interviewing with people with dementia: open-ended interviews probably represent the dominant approach being taken by researchers developing participatory approaches to this point. For example, all but one of the studies reported on in an edited text on research methods involving people with dementia are interview-based studies (Wilkinson, 2002). In addition, interview-based studies are generally sit-down interviews; more spatial methods like walking interviews have yet to become a part of the dementia research toolkit (for a discussion of walking interviews see Emmel and Clark, 2009).

The limitations associated with the use of single source data and straightforward interviewing as a method are already apparent. Increasingly, researchers are experimenting with different media and methods, such as talking mats (Murphy, et al, 2007), the use of video technology and photography to facilitate the interview process. However, while attempts are being made to include the voices of people with dementia, there remains a tendency to still only include those voices that retain the ability to do 'research speak'. In other words, interviews still rely heavily on intact verbal skills even though this is an area that is known to deteriorate with dementia.

One strategy for trying to understand the subjective experience of people with dementia least able to communicate their needs and ideas is through dementia care mapping (DCM). DCM is a structured observation tool that aspires to take the perspective of the person with dementia (Brooker, 2005). The person's state of well-being is documented at five-minute intervals using a 26 behaviour codes list. Although initially designed as a practice tool for understanding resident well-being and examining staff/resident interactions, researchers believe it has the potential as a research instrument (Sloane et al, 2007). The tool is being used internationally – mostly as a practice tool – in 26 different countries. In the UK it is seen as being so useful that a shortened version, known as the short observational framework for inspection (SOFI), has now been designed to assist care home inspectors with their data collection duties in the UK.

Despite its widespread appeal, DCM is not without its critics and methodological limitations. One problem with DCM in the context of this debate is the way it leads researchers to take a non–participatory approach to observation. Generally speaking, the researcher positions themselves at a distance from participants and observes practice against predetermined criteria. In fact, if the person with dementia attempts to interact with the mapper, that five-minute recording period is left blank. Hence, while mappers are trained to be respectful and ethical, there is a clear dividing line that places the person with dementia in a contextual vacuum, vis-à-vis the observation structure. Second, the tool is designed to capture the highest level of well-being. For example, if a person sits glumly for most of the five-minute period, but does smile fleetingly, it is the smiling interaction that would be captured. This may have some tendency to err on the side of overestimating the person's well-being. Third, as highlighted earlier in this book, DCM as a method tends to overlook the wider sociopolitical context in which care actions are taking place. Power differentials between the person giving care and the person receiving that care, and between the caregiver and employer, typically remain unaccounted for. Similarly, the tool does not offer a direct way of taking into account the structural and cultural pressures which an individual caregiver may be experiencing, which may also be preventing them from changing the way they treat a person. An astute mapper may in practice address this in the team discussion that should follow any mapping session, but in research this aspect can get lost.

Although DCM is the best-known form of mapping, there are other ways of mapping that may have potential as a supplement or response to some of these issues. For example, the notion of 'participatory mapping' – an interactive method using adaptable and inventive visual methods (Emmel, 2008) – is creating some excitement among mainstream researchers. The method still involves mapping, of course, but several different types of map can be drawn, for example, social maps, resource maps or a map of a specific issue (like quality of services), and research participants create the maps (not the researchers) in the context of an individual or group interview (Health Development Agency, 2004, p 175).

The point here is that while attempts are being made to involve people with dementia, they require further development and refinement. There is also still room for further imaginative approaches. Figure 6.3 shows some alternative methods of data collection.

Figure 6.3: Some alternative methods of collecting data

Established	Alternative
Dementia care mapping	Ethnographic observations Participant observation Participatory mapping[a]
Sit-down interviews	Walking interviews Walking with video interviews Photo-video diaries
Questionnaires and surveys	Participant-produced video[a] Sound walks Photographic survey Photo or object-elicitation

Note: [a] For further details see the Real Life Methods website, where you will find short documents on the practical aspects of using methods: www.manchester.ac.uk/realities/resources/toolkits

The intention is not to relegate any one particular tool, or to replace one method with another, but to illustrate that other options are available; data do not have to be collected using established methods – other more participatory and creative tools are available and legitimate to use.

Innovative research that recognises the need to extend data generation strategies is being developed. One area of exemplary research practice uses visual data to replace, supplement and/or compliment text-based data to investigate and convey the experience of living with dementia. This work recognises the power and flexibility of a photograph or film to tell a story and employs methods other than interviews to collect data. For example, Cathy Stein Greenblat photographs people with dementia with a view to challenging misconceptions of ageing, ill health and dying (see her website for details of this work at www.cathygreenblat. com/). As Warren and Karner (2005) highlight, Greenblat's choice of method 'gives expression to an experience that could not otherwise be captured and communicated'. Other researchers use cameras and video to collect data, and in so doing provide opportunities for participants to take control and have some fun. For example, Mitchell (2005) conducted a photography project with users of a drop-in centre in Scotland; she asked participants to take photographs of the outings they went on, and then asked them to talk about the images they had taken. Participants reported having a great time and said how much they had learned (about photography) from the project. Hulko (2009) used a similar approach to capture the experiences of people with dementia across different positions of gender, class and ethnicity. Capstick (2009) is engaged in an innovative project using participatory visual methods that takes this one step further. In her study, self-selected members of a day centre use photography, mini-camcorders and online image libraries to tell and share their stories. Visual methods like these recognise that there are other ways, besides language, for understanding the world and people's experiences of it. Moreover, such methods can enable people to participate in a project in an active way and as equals, rather than as 'passive research subjects'.

A second area of alternative research practice uses sound. Researchers in Japan have been working on soundscapes with people with dementia to determine what kinds of sounds are stressful and those that people could easily recollect (Nagahata et al, 2004). The study involved playing a range of environmental sounds, such as kitchen and nature sounds, to men and women with dementia in order to discover how they responded and reacted. Interestingly, the clashing of pots and pans was easily recollected by one woman but represented 'noise' to one of the men.

Research into sound is a growing area of work outside the dementia community. Specifically, researchers in the field of human geography are keen to move away from the idea of negative noise and instead focus on the relevance of positive sounds, like running water and children playing (for details of this work see www. positivesoundscapes.org). Research into sound has the potential to benefit people with dementia, particularly those with low vision and serious sight loss, as it focuses on a critical, but often neglected, aspect of people's experiences – namely aural experience. Moreover, it provides another creative way of generating data that enables participation. In the Positive Soundscape project, for example, participants are asked to go on 'sound walks' where they tell researchers about the sounds they hear and the impact they have on them. In the dementia field, this kind of approach to generating data could really broaden our understanding of how the environment shapes a person's behaviour and well-being.

While these methods are innovative within the dementia field, they are less so within the mainstream qualitative research community where the use of participatory, multisensory methods is becoming more established. Visual methods, in particular, are becoming an increasingly favoured method of collecting data from different social groups including children, people with learning and physical disabilities and those with mental health problems. This is because they allow researchers to investigate the social world in a collaborative and creative way that is more in line with the lives that people are leading (see, for example, Pink, 2007, 2009, and Mason and Davies, 2009, for a more detailed discussion of these issues). The challenge will be for researchers within the dementia community to work in collaboration with researchers from adjacent fields to harness this potential in a way that is relevant and unique to people with dementia.

E: Ethical debates and dilemmas

A social citizenship lens demands a new, more sophisticated examination of the ethical issues underpinning research in the area of dementia. Attention to these issues has already begun to emerge with increasing emphasis being placed on hearing the voice of the person with dementia in research. These issues have mostly centred round issues of 'informed consent' (see, for example, Bartlett and Martin, 2002). One result of these debates has been the call for an 'inclusionary ethical consent process', in which a researcher thinks about and decides how best to involve people with dementia in the research on an ongoing basis (Dewing, 2002, p 168). Strategies for promoting informed consent have included recognising the need to adapt the consent form to accommodate changing cognition. For example, this could include: using simpler language; supplementing words with pictures and/or creating pictorial consent forms; and audio-taping consent rather than relying on written consents. It has also included drawing in notions of procedural consent to accommodate fluctuating memory. This process recognises that willingness and understanding around participation may need to be re-examined repeatedly throughout the process.

Interestingly, while there has been much discussion around the practicalities of gaining informed consent in an ethical way, less emphasis has been placed on how protocols for ensuring informed consent may actually be incongruent with a personhood – let alone citizenship – lens. Arguably, despite legal imperatives that people with dementia are presumed capable, there has been a tendency, especially on the part of behavioural ethics boards, to see people with dementia as 'vulnerable' and hence to err on the side of a more paternalistic approach. For example, in one recent study focused on exploring personhood, in order to meet the requirements of the university ethics committee, the recruitment protocol required that the self-referral by the person with dementia to participate in the study be followed up with a telephone call to the family physician for his/her permission to include that person. The philosophical incongruence of this decision went unchallenged. More commonly, the signature of a family member or 'guardian' is required in addition to that of the person with dementia irrespective of whether or not that person has been found incapable; the assumptions of 'incapacity' hidden behind this practice go unspoken.

The point here is twofold. First, while important inroads have been taken, issues around informed consent are complex and wrought with ambiguity. Further teasing out is still required in order to ensure a sophisticated approach that both recognises citizenship and provides necessary protection. This can be as basic, for example, as considering how a study will be titled on recruitment notices and informed consent forms: how should the references to dementia be made and using what language? The importance of this was brought to light during one recent study. In this study the invitation-to-participate and consent forms recruited 'people with dementia' – a phrase that met ethical requirements of informed consent but caused distress among some potential participants who readily acknowledged memory loss but did not link it to dementia. Some had not been told; others refused to accept the diagnosis. Should we have refused to interview those who did not want to indicate they had dementia but who did indeed want to talk to us about the role of memory loss in their life? Luckily, we were able to find an easy solution that balanced ethical and pragmatic requirements, simply by changing the reference from 'dementia' to 'memory loss' (even while recognising that it too is limited). Each new study, however, raises new questions about how to ensure 'informed consent' without limiting the participation of people who want to contribute.

A second point is to recognise that the informed consent of people with dementia represents only one ethical dilemma in the research process even though discussions of ethical issues have rarely moved beyond this focus into the even murkier area of research ethics. The way in which sometimes even good intentions around promoting personhood and citizenship can result in unanticipated ethical issues is a case in point. For example, in one recent study led by the second co-author (DO), data generation included individual and joint interviews with family members and the person with dementia. The objective was to develop a more comprehensive understanding of the experiences of those using formal support services. While an important piece of this research was to bring in the perspective of the person with dementia as part of the family, it became increasingly apparent that joint interviews often positioned both the person with dementia and the family carer in ways that were distinctly uncomfortable for them. In one interview, for instance, a daughter struggled to present an accurate picture of the situation while simultaneously not challenging her mother's (erroneous) understandings. Sometimes, family members waited until after the interview was over to speak privately with the researcher to provide a different view than that initially presented in the interview; other times they simply spoke over the person with dementia. Irrespective of how this was handled, as researchers we were left feeling uncomfortable and torn. On the one hand, we did not want to talk behind the back of the person with dementia. Worse though were the situations where we watched the undermining of personhood when the family member discounted something that person had said as inaccurate and/or spoke on that person's behalf. We have yet to arrive at the 'right' way of dealing with this. Is it our role to intervene when we see disrespectful practice occurring? If so, what are the ethical implications of silencing often very well-meaning and stressed family members (and what are the pragmatic implications of this on our research if we do so)?

The main point here then is that practitioners engaged in research-related activities that reflect a social citizenship value lens will be called on to make choices and sometimes difficult decisions about a range of ethical issues before, during and after the research process. These include, for example, how to:

- judge and enable a level of participation that is right for each participant;
- distinguish between protection, paternalism and care;
- negotiate and gain permission to use cameras, videos and other recording devices, particularly in medical settings;
- manage relational dynamics (for example, between the gatekeeper, research participant, spouse, and other family members);
- educate members of ethics committee, and others, about the dangers of making assumptions about people with dementia.

C: Critical lens

Just over 10 years ago Kitwood and others urged researchers to investigate the subjective experiences of people with dementia. A number of ways were suggested in order to do this, including, for example, talking to people with dementia, listening attentively to what they had to say and reading biographical accounts (Kitwood, 1997b). Since then researchers, practitioners, governments and charitable organisations have all endeavoured to find out more about the lived experience of dementia (see, for example, Alzheimer's Society, 2008; Phinney, 2008). This has been an important area of research. It has given people with dementia a voice and helped others to gain more insight into people's abilities and experiences. It has certainly challenged a tendency to envision the person with dementia as being entirely subsumed by it.

While research into personal experience has proved influential in drawing attention to the shared everyday realities that cut across individual lives, accounts are often accepted uncritically, with little attention given to power dynamics and wider contextual factors; hence the emphasis shifts towards helping the individual 'cope' with dementia, rather than on what needs to change in society to promote social citizenship. For example, the degree to which a person's account of living with dementia reflects broader societal oppressive discourses (such as ageism and racism) is rarely open to scrutiny. Moreover, focusing only on the subjective experience of dementia fails to recognise either the capacity or desire of individuals to look beyond themselves and their own issues. Some researchers have attempted to link these individualised accounts to broader societal responses, but this has not been the dominant approach (see, for example, Hulko, 2009;

O'Connor et al, 2009). The problem is that collective experiences are overlooked or lost when the emphasis is on the individual; this in turn perpetuates the view that the experience of disability 'stems from the individual', as opposed to society (Moore et al, 1998, p 12).

In order to gain a richer, more contextualised understanding of the issues facing people with dementia, research that draws on critical theories and research methodologies that allow for investigation into, and analysis of, the interplay between subjective experience and sociopolitical and cultural context, is required. There are a variety of ways that this can be done. We will highlight four approaches that have particular relevance in dementia studies: narrative techniques, institutional ethnography, Foucauldian methods and Bourdieu's sociological approach to research. We note that this is not an exhaustive range of routes; rather the intent is simply to open for discussion the possibilities for seeing beyond immediate experience.

Narrative techniques

Narrative techniques are gaining in popularity as an approach to research with people with dementia. Narrative techniques seek 'to interpret the ways in which people perceive reality, make sense of their worlds, and perform social actions' (Phoenix et al, 2010, p 4). A key principle when using narrative techniques is to keep the process of data generation sufficiently flexible so that it can generate 'stories'. Often this translates into the value of more unstructured ways of generating data that give the person with dementia control and authority over what gets said and relayed, and how it gets said and relayed.

This approach is being used with increasing frequency in research with people with dementia. (Keady et al, 2005, for example, have done exemplary work in this area using narrative methods.) To date, the transcripts that develop from this approach have typically been analysed from a more phenomenological perspective with the goal of developing in-depth insight into the subjective experiences and perspectives of the person with dementia. This has been absolutely critical for expanding understanding of the dementia experiences. However, as outlined earlier in this book, this approach is not necessarily conducive to an analysis that extends to the interplay between subjective experience and sociopolitical and cultural context.

Narrative techniques that draw on discourse analytic strategies allow this same data to be analysed in a way that fosters an understanding of this interplay. There are a variety of ways for conducting discourse analysis that lead to a focus beyond the individual narrative. Generally, however, when used to elicit the link between subjective experiences and sociopolitical context, three broad assumptions ground the importance of personal stories. First, consistent with narrative approaches in general, texts and stories are used to conceptualise the ways in which individuals develop systems of meanings and beliefs; people not only interpret, but actually organise their experiences through storying and performing those stories (Bruner,

1987). Second, personal stories are organised according to culturally available but tacit 'reasoning' procedures (Widdicombe, 1993); culture speaks through an individual's story (Rosenwald and Ochberg, 1992; Daiute and Lightfoot, 2004). This means that the personal story reflects the beliefs, ideas and messages to which a person has been exposed as they have interacted with their familial, political, social, economic, spiritual and cultural milieus. Thus, the third assumption is that the analysis of the texts of personal narratives makes visible not only the individual's experience but also helps to contextualise that experience within a broader sociocultural context. From a political perspective, this analysis can be used to comment on social processes that participate in the maintenance of structures of oppression (Kvale, 1996). Hence, a discourse analysis implicitly adopts a critical standpoint that challenges taken-for-granted assumptions.

There are a few examples of this approach in the area of dementia studies. For instance, O'Connor et al (2009) use this approach to understand how the discourses associated with the social location of an aboriginal, middle-aged, lesbian woman with vascular dementia conspired and worked both together, and in opposition, to construct a personal experience that was individually unique but obviously shaped by broader societal discourses. This analysis revealed the tension and points of contradiction between at least four different discourses (biomedical, aboriginal, heterosexism and ageism) as they impacted on this woman's day-to-day experiences of living with dementia.

Narrative research is important because it facilitates a contextualising of dementia experiences that captures complexity, contradictions and diversity while retaining a solid grounding in the personal experiences of the individual. Within the field of dementia research there already exists a growing body of stories by and for people with dementia. These stories provide the link between individual experiences and broader sociopolitical and cultural contexts. Research examining them within this light will be an important next step.

Institutional ethnography

A second route to investigating the interplay between experience and sociopolitical context is through institutional ethnography. This approach to research seeks to understand the standpoint, or subject position, of a particular group by seeking to uncover the '"ruling relations" – that is, those extraordinary yet ordinary set of relations that are textually mediated, and connect us across space and time and organise our everyday lives – the corporations, government bureaucracies, academic and professional discourses, mass media and the complex of relations that interconnect them' (Smith, 2005, p 10). As further described by Smith (2005), institutional ethnography:

> ... is a method of inquiry that begins with the actualities of people's everyday lives and experiences and seeks to discover the social as it extends beyond this experience.... The institutional ethnographer

works from the social in people's experience to discover its presence and organization in their lives and to explicate or map that organization beyond the local of the everyday. (pp 10-11)

This form of ethnography seeks to discover how 'ruling relations' or organisational practices and policies construct and shape personal experience. It involves the researcher taking a critical stance and 'reaching beyond local particularities of people's everyday lives and into the regions of the relations that organise them' (Smith, 2005, pp 57/8). So, as well as investigating individual experience and actions, the institutional ethnographer seeks to uncover the wider organisational processes and systems in which they are embedded and played out. For example, a research team might decide to take the standpoint of women with dementia, not because women are biologically different from men, but because, as a social group, women have different experiences of men due to the gendered nature of the labour market.

Within the field of dementia studies, there are one or two examples of research that have taken this approach. For example, a study by McColgan (2005) focused on people with dementia in nursing homes. She discovered that where residents sat was a source of struggle and that the organisational practice of changing seating arrangements was an inextricable part of that experience:

> Selecting a place to sit and creating defensible space around it was one way in which [residents] could [exercise autonomy and choice]. However, the rearrangement of furniture [by staff] often denied this choice and made the place unfamiliar and without areas of defence. (McColgan, 2005, p 430)

This exemplar demonstrates the point of an institutional ethnography: linking micro experiences with institutional process is a useful way of discovering not only more about individual experience but also the power and influence of social systems and relations. While there are other examples of research related to dementia studies taking this kind of approach (see, for example, Diamond, 1992; Proctor, 2001), this approach to research in the field of dementia studies remains under-developed and mostly limited in its focus to long-term care. With the recent emphasis on research that attempts to capture the perspective – or 'standpoint' – of people with dementia the first step in developing an institutional ethnography has been taken. The next step is to recognise this insight as a 'point of entry' (Smith, 2005 p 10) into wider social investigation and move beyond individual experience.

Foucauldian methods

A third promising methodological route for forging the link between the subjective and the social can be found in the ideas of French philosopher Michel Foucault (1926–84). Foucault was interested in the historical origins of power. He wrote extensively about how power is (re)produced in different social institutions, such as hospitals, asylums and prisons, and through cultural mechanisms such as the (re)production of knowledge. An important thesis underlying Foucault's work is that any given system of thought or practice is the accumulation of past events and therefore contingent on history. In other words, what happens now is inextricably connected to the past. For example, the housing of people with dementia within care homes, and especially placing people with advanced dementia in a 'dementia wing', which is usually upstairs, arguably dates back to the long-term (disabling) practice of using space to segregate people with disabilities from the rest of society (Kitchin, 1998). Foucauldian methods focus attention on how subjective experiences are inextricably linked to the historical (re)production(s) of power.

Brijnath and Manderson (2008) provide one example of research conducted in the area of dementia studies using Foucauldian methods. The research was conducted in India and identifies and describes the significance of three historical power/knowledge scripts in the context of long-term care, namely: social and cultural notions of acceptable public bodies; medicalised forms of care; and the cultural contexts of the individual caregivers. They conclude that:

> ... the caregiver is the embodiment of these discourses and is charged with the task of mapping discipline onto inherently undisciplinable bodies. A tension exists between caregiver's struggle to contain the unruliness of the person with dementia and, simultaneously, to act as a broker between the world of the care-recipient and the social world.... [A]lthough the caregiver is the starting point for the exercise of discipline, the three power/knowledge scripts that inform care work areas are as much about surveying, routinizing and mobilizing caregivers' bodies as they are about disciplining the bodies of people with dementia. (Brijnath and Manderson, 2008, p 607)

Through their work they strive to complicate the mind–body dualism, arguing that the power that people with dementia have is not rooted in their mind or soul or sense of self, as Descartes originally proposed; nor is it realised by attribution from other people, as Kitwood theorised. Rather, the power that people with dementia have is in their bodies (Brijnath and Manderson, 2008). Their work provides an interesting example on how research can move beyond the taken-for-granted to reveal new ways of understanding and challenging existing status quo.

Drawing on Bourdieu

A fourth exciting way of making this link is beginning to emerge through work that is drawing on the ideas of the French sociologist Pierre Bourdieu (1930-2002). Like Foucault, Bourdieu saw the social world as the accumulation of history; however, Bourdieu took as his starting point the individual, and in particular, the agency or capacity of an individual to engage with the social world. Bourdieu developed the notion of habitus to explain and understand how individuals interact with and make sense of the social world in which they live. The notion of habitus is integral to Bourdieu's work and can be defined as 'a subjective, internal construction, an experience of everyday life, in a dialectical relationship with the wider world' (Gauntlett, 2007, p 64). It captures the way in which our stories and actions, our lives, are inextricably linked to and accumulated through societal practices and customs.

Smith (2009) provides an example of using Bourdieu to conceptualise issues of capacity in dementia. He suggests that Bourdieu 'challenges us to think about the relations of domination between individuals and their social institutions' (p 42), and hence has important implications for analysing the ongoing power relations between individuals diagnosed with dementia and the institutions mandated to evaluate their cognitive capacity. In his analysis, he interrogates the discourses of dementia that privilege individualising notions of capacity, autonomy and independence, and calls for a more culturally contextualised approach to analysing experience. Kontos (2004, 2005) similarly uses a Bourdieu analysis in her research to demonstrate an embodied self-hood in dementia, or using Bourdieu-speak, an embodied cultural capital that remains long after verbal skills have deteriorated.

When drawing on Bourdieu, it is important to remember that 'a person's agency is heavily prescribed by the social circumstances in which they find themselves' (Gauntlett, 2007, p 67). Moreover, a person's circumstances will differ depending on the forms of capital that they possess or have access to. According to Bourdieu, there are two principal forms of capital, namely, cultural and social capital. Both forms of capital manifest in different ways, for example, cultural capital can take the form of actual cultural goods (such as books, works of art) or it can be more embodied in form (such as being able to use technologies and digilocks, or knowing how to access services) (Bourdieu, 1986). In contrast, social capital refers to the resources that a person has; these might be social resources (such as colleagues, friends and neighbours) or they might be material resources (such as money, means of private transport, gadgets). From Bourdieu's perspective, the important point is that there are many forms of capital, not just wealth.

In order to show how the ideas of Bourdieu might be drawn to expand dementia research, it might be helpful to look at and (re)analyse some existing text. The text selected is from the work of the poet John Killick, who takes the exact words and phrases of people with dementia and reconstructs them in the form of a poem:

> It's really scary when you're an old woman.
> I'm bereft. I hate being stranded like this,
> I want to go down in the middle of town.
> But I have no money to speak of, and
> I don't know how to get away from here.
> I can't open it! The door won't open. (Killick and Allan, 2001, p 272)

By using poetic conventions the experience of care home life for this woman is powerfully portrayed (Bartlett, 2004, p 31). The issue is, it is then analysed in the context of loss and bereavement without reference to the wider sociopolitical context, and so a fuller understanding is not gained. If you were drawing on Bourdieu, an alternative reading of this poem might look something like this:

Comment	Might suggest a lack of
'It's really scary when you're an old woman.	(social status)
I'm bereft. I hate being stranded like this,	(cultural capital)
I want to go down in the middle of town	(access to transportation)
But I have no money to speak of, and	(economic capital)
I don't know how to get away from here	(cultural capital, specifically local knowledge)
I can't open it! The door won't open.	(embodied cultural capital)

Thus by drawing on Bourdieu, particularly the notions of habitus and capital, a different, extremely useful way of thinking about a person's situation begins to emerge. No longer is it just about personal loss and bereavement but also social (im)position and lack of resources.

Summary

Narrative research, institutional ethnography, Foucauldian methods and drawing on Bourdieu – the message underlying all these routes is not to stop at subjective experience. As Czarniawska says (2004, p 5), 'we are never the sole author of our own narratives', there will always be other factors at play – whether they be: competing stories (narrative analysis); ruling relations and systems (institutional ethnography); historical power dynamics (Foucauldian methods); or social location and capital (drawing on Bourdieu) – something will always be entwining with and shaping our subjective experience. The challenge for researchers is to identify and disentangle those influences, and to retell people's stories in a way that is fully contextualised.

Each of the routes described in this chapter demonstrates the possibilities that are emerging for creatively using critical research methodology to examine the link between the personal and social. Unquestionably, there are other useful routes. The point is to highlight the need for research to move beyond more phenomenologically oriented approaches for understanding experiences in order to begin to critically position people with dementia within a broader sociopolitical context. Research approaches grounded in critical theory offer exciting opportunities for beginning to consider and conceptualise this link.

T: Translation of research into practice

We begin this section by identifying the importance of research for developing new knowledge and approaches to practice – creating 'evidence'. Alongside this growing emphasis on the importance of evidence-based practice is the recognition that to be useful, research must be used. This in turn has led to centring the importance of knowledge translation and exchange activities as an essential part of the research process: funding bodies, even those considered more academic, are increasingly demanding that proposals for research funding include a section outlining a feasible plan for reaching key stakeholders and ensuring uptake of the research. Using terminology such as 'knowledge to action', 'knowledge transfer' or 'knowledge translation and exchange' – rather than the conventional dissemination – a new body of literature is beginning to emerge outlining effective approaches for ensuring that research is both useable and used.

A key principles underpinning much of this developing body of literature is that learning is social – people learn in practice, by doing and interacting with others – and knowledge exchange can be empowering and lead to social change. One way that this may be done is by challenging traditional hierarchical ways of delivering education/support and adapting more liberating practices (Freire, 1985) that recognise the expertise that people with dementia and family members continue to bring into the situation. Drawing on the ideas associated with Freire's critical pedagogy, if knowledge is to be empowering, it must: (a) recognise the connection between what is being learned and a person's overall life experiences; (b) position all learners as 'experts' in some field of their own lives; and (c) engage participants as active, rather than passive, consumers. This approach also recognises learning and knowledge production as inherently social. It is within this social context that individuals are able to reframe their individual troubles as public issues, not personal deficiencies. This step, particularly when it occurs within the context of a validating community, creates the context for social action and empowerment.

These ideas are directly in line with a social citizenship approach, which demands the unsettling of power relationships between consumers (person with dementia and family care partners) and professionals (including researchers, policy and practice leaders and front-line care staff); challenging the individualisation of issues; and creating an opportunity for people with dementia and their care partners to influence the various communities in which they interact, including the research community.

As one approach for achieving this, Phinney (2008) proposes a three-principled framework for considering effective knowledge translation with people with dementia: adaptation, dialogue and advocacy. Adaptation takes into account that the cognitive impairments related to dementia require adapting how information is provided. For example, this means considering the use of different channels for presenting information about research findings – innovative researchers are successfully using strategies such as life theatre and drama, visual methods such as photographic displays, creative writing (including poems) and video and audio-tracks that are website accessible. Others are using more conventional ways, but adapting these to accommodate memory changes. These approaches are exciting and promising.

The second principle, dialogue, recognises the social nature of learning – people learn better when they engage in conversations rather than simply having knowledge passed down to them. Thus, one effective strategy for disseminating research-based knowledge is the strategic use of the group context. Groups provide a community context for countering the stigma and demoralisation that people with dementia and their family live with on a day-to-day basis, and can foster a sense of competence, connection and citizenship. Furthermore, there is power in numbers: presenting research findings within a group context ensures that the researcher is outnumbered, which in some ways may help to offset traditional power dynamics that are often inherent in the researcher/researched relationship.

The third principle, advocacy, is particularly relevant within the context of social citizenship. Specifically, this process recognises that people with dementia, including existing groups such as DASNI and SDWG, are in excellent positions to assist in getting research out through personal and political networks. This is both empowering – they control the information that is passed on – and effective.

New knowledge gained through research has the potential to change how we think about people with dementia and can change people's experiences with dementia. However, it is only useful when it is actually used to inform practice and experiences. A critical ingredient of a social citizenship approach to research practice then requires careful and creative exploration of ways to ensure that this translation of research speak to lay speak actually occurs and occurs in a way that is empowering.

Conclusion

Research grounded in the ideas of social citizenship is explicitly political, broader in vision and recognises the rights of people with dementia to participate in meaningful and equal ways in the development of knowledge that is relevant and useful to them. Using the EXPECT framework, this chapter has argued for a more thoughtful, imaginative and contextualised vision in terms of agenda setting and methodological choices than is currently practiced in the dementia field. It has sought to raise awareness of the narrowness of the current research agenda and has highlighted some of the methodological limitations of popular tools, including DCM. Proposals have been made for new topics to research, which would radically expand knowledge and provide opportunities for people with dementia to control and fully participate in the research process. Further, the chapter has called for more creativity and sensitivity in terms of approach and choice of methods. Underpinning this discussion has been the implicit assumption that there are multiple ways of knowing (some are sensorial or tacit) that interview and observations methods cannot access or ascertain, and so individual researchers must use and develop sensory and participatory approaches to research. By engaging in the methods and approaches outlined in this chapter, the dementia research community can move towards a more critical citizenship-based approach to social research.

Note
[1] For further information about this project contact the Arts Development Officer at Wigan Leisure & Culture Trust, Elizabeth House, The Pier, Wigan WN3 4BD.

Part III
Combining theory and practice

SEVEN

Conclusion: working towards social citizenship

Introduction

Understanding of dementia has evolved considerably over the past few decades, from considering serious cognitive impairment as an expectable part of the ageing process, to recognising dementia as a biomedical phenomenon, and then towards the importance of seeing beyond the bio-physiological issues to the person behind the label. It is time for the emergence of a fourth moment: centring dementia experiences, as shaped and constrained by broader sociopolitical systems, discourses and life events.

The aim of this book has been to broaden the dementia debate by outlining an approach that can take understanding and practice into this fourth moment. It has considered the situation of people with dementia from an explicitly sociopolitical perspective and identified and discussed issues beyond health and social care. Discussion has highlighted the narrowness of the current agenda in the dementia field and aimed to raise the stakes in terms of thinking about the status, experiences, responsibilities and entitlements of men and women with dementia. It has sought to reposition people as active citizens, as opposed to only welfare recipients, and to show the contribution people with dementia can and do make to everyday life. Simultaneously, it has argued the need to revise understanding of social citizenship in order to account for neuro-cognitive changes that may interfere with conventional participation and involvement.

We acknowledge that there are undoubtedly limitations and deficiencies in our thinking and that some of the ideas explored in this book are in their infancy, and arguably quite radical for this field. In particular, we accept that in certain circumstances ideas about social citizenship might jar with other key debates in the field, including, for example, those around safeguarding vulnerable adults and balancing the rights of people with dementia with the rights of others. Enabling the social citizenship of people with dementia is a complex area and this book is recognised as only a start to the discussion. We have tentatively aimed to open up debate about people with dementia in order to explicitly consider another aspect of people's situation.

In this conclusion we will draw together the dominant themes that underpin this book and highlight some of the key messages that the field might take forward. The discussion is organised around three key points: (1) the importance of bringing a sociopolitical perspective to the fore; (2) the relevance of a social citizenship lens for elevating status and recognition of a more dynamic, politically informed understanding of dementia; and (3) the importance of seeing beyond the care context. The remainder of this chapter summarises key messages and identifies ways to move forward in each of these three areas. Our hope is to leave the reader with a renewed vision and sense of purpose in terms of finding ways to support and work with people with dementia. Further, it is anticipated that dialogue about the utility and meaning of citizenship for the dementia field will be stimulated.

Bringing a sociopolitical perspective to the fore

Unlike most other texts in the field this book has prioritised the importance of contextualising personal and interpersonal experiences of dementia within a broader sociopolitical and cultural dimension. Our intention has not been to relegate or undermine psychological (nor indeed neurological) constructs but rather to add a more sociological-oriented perspective that draws attention to how experiences and actions are shaped and constrained by societal structures, systems and discourses in order that broader dynamics might be revealed and debated. Our argument has been that attempts to understand both psychosocial and neurological issues in a vacuum result in an incomplete picture that disadvantages people with dementia.

We are not unique in identifying the need to bring sociopolitical issues to the fore, however. It has been on the agenda for some time. For example, early work by Bond (1992) and Herskovits (1995) certainly set the stage for this vision. Shortly after, Cantley and Bowes (2004, p 269) argued that we should 'think in terms of ensuring people's rights as citizens as well as their personhood; and in terms of community development and political activism as well as service development'. This book has sought to contribute to and advance this work in a theoretically informed way but also to extend this debate to envision new practices.

In bringing sociopolitical issues to the fore, a different range of issues has come under the spotlight. These include, for example, the importance of recognising the emergence of community spirit and connections between citizens with dementia. Until now debate has generally focused on relations between caregivers and individuals with dementia; with few exceptions, little attention has been paid to relations between people with dementia (Clare et al, 2008). In a way the relationships people with dementia have with each other have been invisible in scholarly debate. When these relationships are considered, it is often within the context of emotional support rather than community action and solidarity. This book has sought to extend dialogue by highlighting how peer support and solidarity might be achieved in more informal ways.

Importantly, the focus on sociopolitical issues brings to the forefront the issue of power, not just the power of caregivers and service providers but also, and more critically, the power – or lack of power – of men and women with dementia. Throughout this book, examples have been given to highlight the individual and collective efforts of people with dementia to fight stigma and discrimination, as well as the capacity of individuals through vignettes and discussions to assert their rights and political voice. We have then looked at how approaches to practice and research might foster the retention of power, or at least avoid disempowering. Prioritising sociopolitical issues, such as power and agency, raises the stakes in terms of conceptualising the status, experiences and entitlements of people with dementia. It also expands the imagination in practice and social research.

Coming at dementia from a sociopolitical angle raises practical, as well as conceptual, issues. An important focus of this book has been on the applied value of a sociopolitical perspective. It has shown how taking a sociopolitical perspective has important implications for practitioners and researchers alike. For example, in Chapter Six some imaginative ways of enabling participation in research were proposed and discussed. Wherever possible, and particularly in Part II, discussion has focused on what a sociopolitical perspective might mean in an applied and everyday sense.

It is recognised there are inherent dangers with bringing sociopolitical issues to the fore. One of the potential risks is that internal factors are negated as external factors are taken to be the dominant influence in a person's life. In the same way that there is a risk of 'over-psychologising' the individual – that is, of seeing everything at a micro/internal level – there is a risk of 'over-socialising' the individual as well – everything is seen as having an external cause. Clarke and Marshall (2001) are scholars who seek to bring a sociopolitical perspective to the fore in their field and discuss this problem in relation to older people's experiences of stroke. These authors suggest that one way around the above dilemma is to ensure that both perspectives are simultaneously taken into account. The challenge in dementia studies will be to recognise the need to do this, and to establish this balance.

Lastly, bringing a sociopolitical perspective to the fore serves to enrich and deepen the story about the situation of people with dementia. To date only certain parts of the 'dementia story' have been fully told, namely, the scientific/ neurological and psychosocial parts. By introducing a sociopolitical perspective into the debate a fuller, more relational story about people's experiences of dementia can be considered. The advantage here is that this points to ways that society as a whole must change, rather than assuming change can only occur at an individual or micro level.

Using social citizenship to elevate status and understanding

At the start of this book we discussed the intractable problem of low status. Attention to personhood has dominated professional discourse as a core concept for tackling this since the early 1990s. While important, it is not sufficiently inclusive or expansive enough to capture the full range of individual and collective needs and rights of people with dementia; it may not be the best lens for capturing the full spectrum of people's situations. As has been shown in this book, men and women with dementia are an extremely heterogeneous social group. Some individuals will have enjoyed a lifetime of wealth and privilege, whereas others will have encountered hardship or discrimination. Added to this, dementia is an illness that can affect anybody at virtually any time during the adult lifecourse and so there will inevitably be intergenerational differences in terms of lived experience and status.

Social citizenship emerges as an important concept for fostering a more comprehensive discussion. Where personhood is an intuitively appealing concept, citizenship is a more challenging term that conjures up a different set of issues, issues that revolve around notions of entitlement, power, status and responsibilities. Arguably, it is a more far-reaching term, and provides the language for thinking about people's experiences and status in a fundamentally different way.

At a most basic level, attention to citizenship points to a different set of questions. Why, for example, has dementia had such poor status in relation to other disabling conditions? A citizenship lens draws attention to the existing trend to privilege the experiences of people with physical impairment, both in theory and practice, over those with a cognitive impairment (Seddon et al, 2001). It is not clear why people with dementia should be overlooked within the broader disability studies field. One possible explanation is that this field is dominated by younger people, usually men, with a physical (as opposed to cognitive) disability (Adams and Bartlett, 2003). Another might be that disability scholars are simply not interested in dementia-related issues, perhaps reflective of the ageist society in which we live. Thus the notion of citizenship draws attention to the marginalised status of people with dementia across disability discourse as a whole, and facilitates a critical analysis that draws attention to how systems of discrimination – including sexism, ageism, racism and ableism – may work in tandem.

This book has opened the dementia field up to discourses about citizenship. We have drawn on the work of critical social citizenship theorists to begin to develop a more embedded conceptualisation of citizenship. For example, one important focus has been to use the concept of citizenship strategically to critique, problematise and extend some of the ideas that have so far largely gone unchallenged in the field, including, for example, the ideas of 'comfort', 'attachment', 'occupation', inclusion', 'identity' and 'love'. A more culturally dynamic understanding is promoted that attends to issues such as purpose, participation, social positions, community and discrimination. The aim is not to replace existing concepts but to show how the field might benefit from using constructs from citizenship studies in order to expand the imagination and adopt a more active approach to understanding and responding to people with dementia.

While there are clearly advantages to using citizenship as an organising framework, several problems arise when it is used in relation to people with dementia. One is that because citizenship is so closely associated with responsibility and civic duties, it can be seen as placing undue and unrealistic demands on some individuals – how can a very frail older person with advanced dementia be an active citizen and fulfil civic duties such as voting? Similarly, what meaning can the idea of a 'responsible citizen' have in relation to people who are at the very end stages of their life? The idea of passive citizenship, discussed in Chapter Three, helps to address this problem to some extent – people who are very cognitively impaired are entitled to welfare, rather than expected to take on responsibilities. However, even here the fundamental issue of there being a conceptual link between citizenship and responsibility remains unaddressed. One possible way around this issue is to think in terms of the fluidity of responsibility – that is to say, rather than seeing it as a hard and fixed set task (such as voting), see it in degrees and in terms of shifting expectations. In practice, that would mean inviting and expecting people to take on as much or as little responsibility as they can handle. This is certainly an area that requires further discussion.

Clearly, attention to rights and responsibilities, and the practice of citizenship, must be understood within the context of a disease process that interferes with intellectual functioning. Thus, the argument that dementia must be contextualised within the broader sociopolitical context is too one-sided. Offsetting it is the counter-argument that the socio-political context, captured under the umbrella of social citizenship, must be contextualised within the realities of dementia. In other words, meaning and ideals underpinning traditional notions of citizenship must be renegotiated in the context of dementia.

A second problem relates to implementation of the equality principle. What precisely does this mean and how can it be operationalised in a way that also recognises differences, especially in relation to cognitive abilities? If we are to say that a person with dementia must be treated as an equal citizen, is it not logical to then say that that person should be punished or reprimanded in the same way as any other citizen, as and when they transgress social and cultural norms (such as waking neighbours at night, taking other people's belongings and so forth)? Similarly, some might argue that it follows that people with dementia should be expected to fulfil their obligations as citizens in the same way as everybody else. These are thorny and complex issues, which this book has raised rather than answered.

Clearly using citizenship to raise the status of people with dementia is an important area for further development, and this book has raised many questions for debate. In particular, one of the areas that we continue to grapple with is the relationship between personhood and citizenship. What does this look like and how does it change as the dementia advances? Conceivably the importance of each aspect of the experience may ebb and flow depending on both the individual experiences and the degree of neuropathological change. Other important questions the book raises are:

• What limits and enhances people's ability to practise as citizens?
• How useful is the concept of citizenship to dementia care practice?
• To what extent is the concept of citizenship in synchrony with the value base of other cultures?

- How congruent do practitioners find the concept of citizenship to creating an enabling culture?

These are important questions not only for dementia studies but also for wider disability and citizenship studies discourse.

Seeing beyond care

The routine pairing of dementia with care, as in reference to 'dementia care', captures the implicit prioritising of a care focus in dementia studies. In particular, the unspoken and unexplored assumption is that people with dementia can only be understood and responded to as welfare recipients, or at least in relation to a care discourse. An important theme underpinning this book is the need to go beyond care issues and to see men and women with dementia in a much more contextualised and dynamic way – as a highly diverse group of people with the ability to affect as well as to be affected.

This has potentially huge implications pragmatically. Primarily, it means that people are seen as having multiple social positions, as opposed to that of simply a care recipient. We begin to notice and appreciate the other social identities a person with dementia might have, not just their identity as a 'care recipient', including, for example:

- activist
- advocate
- author
- artist
- blogger
- campaigner
- educator/trainer
- employee
- friend/confidant
- fundraiser
- lover
- public speaker
- taxpayer
- theist
- volunteer
- voter.

This list is obviously not exhaustive. The critical point is that by looking beyond the welfare context, a more equitable way of thinking and talking about people with dementia begins to emerge. The 'them' and 'us' barrier is challenged, and a more dynamic understanding emerges which recognises that all people can simultaneously occupy multiple social positions including, but not limited to, that of someone with care needs.

We are sensitive to the counter-argument that care has a vital role to play in the lives of many people with dementia, particularly those who are severely cognitively impaired, and/or who have other health conditions. Clearly care is an important component in all our lives, and it has therefore not been suggested in this book that sociopolitical constructs replace concepts of care. To the contrary, questions have been raised regarding the implicit positioning of someone who needs care in a way that devalues them. We have highlighted how societal assumptions about care and receiving care serve to disadvantage people with dementia. We hope the case has been made for a more critical approach to care.

Seeing beyond care challenges how we practise, opening up new ways of working with people with dementia that do not necessarily position people only as clients needing help. It highlights gaps in research that need to be addressed, especially highlighting how little we actually know about other aspects of people's lives including work and use of services such as transportation and leisure. It also merges with ongoing concern about the narrow homogenised understanding we have so far developed around dementia, reiterating that we need to understand people's experiences within a lifecourse perspective, one which attends to notions of social location, in order to develop a more textured, and useful, understanding of dementia.

Finally, the aim of this book has been to expand imagination in the dementia debate. We have sought to raise questions and awareness, and to inform and provoke debate, rather than to provide definitive answers or solutions. Our discussion has been deliberately consciousness-raising rather than prescriptive in tone; we have neither the desire nor capacity to impose a particular framework or way of thinking on practice. That said, we hope that the issues raised will at least inspire those working in the field to think even more deeply and critically about the social and research practices they engage in. It may even propel some into taking positive action.

References

Adams, T. (1996) 'Kitwood's approach to dementia and dementia care: a critical but appreciative review', *Journal of Advanced Nursing*, 23: 949-53.

Adams, T. and Bartlett, R. (2003) 'Constructing dementia', in T. Adams and J. Manthorpe (eds) (2003) *Dementia Care*, London: Arnold Publishers.

Alzheimer's Society (2008) *Dementia: Out of the shadows*, London: Alzheimer's Society.

Arnstein, S. (1969) 'A ladder of citizen participation', *Journal of the American Institute of Planners*, vol 35, no 4, pp 216-24.

Baldwin, C. (2008) 'Narrative (,) Citizenship and dementia: The personal and the political', *Journal of Aging Studies*, vol 22, 3, pp 222-28.

Baldwin, C. and Capstick, A. (eds) (2007) *Tom Kitwood on dementia: A reader and critical commentary*, Maidenhead: McGraw-Hill/Open University Press.

Banerjee, S. (2009) *The use of antipsychotic medication for people with dementia: Time for action. A Report for the Minister of State for Care Services by Professor Sube Banerjee*, (Available to download from www.dh.gov.uk/en/Publicationsandstatistics/Publications/PublicationsPolicyAndGuidance/DH_108303).

Barnes, C., Mercer, G. and Shakespeare, T. (1999) *Exploring disability: A sociological introduction*, Cambridge: Polity Press (in association with Blackwell Publishers Ltd).

Barnes, M. (1997) *Care, communities and citizens*, London: Longman.

Barnes, M. and Brannelly, T. (2008) 'Achieving care and social justice for people with dementia', *Nursing Ethics*, vol 15, no 3, pp 384-95.

Barnes, R., Auburn, T. and Lea, S. (2004) 'Citizenship in practice', *British Journal of Social Psychology*, vol 43, pp 187-206.

Barnett, E. (2000) *Including the person with dementia in designing and delivering care: "I need to be me!"*, London: Jessica Kingsley Publishers.

Bartlett, H. and Martin, W. (2002) 'Ethical issues in dementia care research', in H. Wilkinson (ed) *The perspectives of people with dementia: Research methods and motivations*, London: Jessica Kingsley Publishers, pp 47-63.

Bartlett, R. (2004) 'Meanings of social exclusion and inclusion in relation to older people with dementia in care homes', Unpublished PhD thesis, Oxford Brookes University.

Bartlett, R. (2007) '"You can get in alright, but you can't get out": social exclusion and men with dementia in care homes', *Quality in Ageing: Policy, Practice and Research*, vol 8, no 2, pp 16-26.

Bartlett, R. and O'Connor, D. (2007) 'From personhood to citizenship: broadening the lens for dementia practice and research', *Journal of Aging Studies*, vol 21, pp 107-18.

Bates, J., Boote, J. and Beverley, C. (2004) 'Psychosocial interventions for people with a milder dementing illness: a systematic review', *Journal of Advanced Nursing*, vol 45, no 6, pp 644-58.

Bauman, Z. (1992) *Imitations of postmodernity*, London: Routledge.

BBC (2007) 'Alzheimer's drugs remain limited', Friday, 10 August 2007 (http://news.bbc.co.uk/1/low/health/6939950.stm).

Beard, R. (2004) 'Advocating voice: organisational, historical and social milieux of the Alzheimer's disease movement', *Sociology of Health and Illness*, vol 26, no 6, pp 797-819.

Bender, M. and Cheston, R. (1997) 'Inhabitants of a Lost Kingdom: a model of the subjective experiences of dementia', *Ageing and Society*, vol 17, pp 513-32.

Bickel, A. (1975) *The morality of consent*, New Haven, CT, and London: Yale University Press.

Bond, J. (1992) 'The medicalisation of dementia', *Journal of Aging Studies*, vol 92, no 6(4), pp 397-403.

Bond, J., Corner, L. and Graham, R. (2004) 'Social science theory on dementia research: normal ageing, cultural representation and social exclusion', in A. Innes, C. Archibald and C. Murphy (eds) *Dementia and social inclusion: Marginalised groups and marginalised areas of dementia research, care and practice*, London: Jessica Kingsley Publishers, pp 220-37.

Booth, T. and Booth, W. (1996) 'Sounds of silence: narrative research with inarticulate subjects', *Disability & Society*, vol 11, no 1, pp 55-69.

Bourdieu, P. (1986) 'The forms of capital', in J. Richardson (ed) *Handbook of theory and research for the sociology of education*, New York, NY: Greenwood, pp 241-58.

Bowlby, J. (1979) *The making and breaking of affectional bonds*, London: Tavistock.

Boyle, G. (2008) 'The Mental Capacity Act 2005: promoting the citizenship of people with dementia?', *Health and Social Care in the Community*, vol 16, no 5, pp 529-37.

Bracken, P. and Thomas, P. (2005) *Postpsychiatry*, Oxford: Oxford University Press.

Braudy-Harris, P. (ed) (2002a) *The person with Alzheimer's disease: Pathways to understanding the experience*, Baltimore, MD and London: The John Hopkins University Press.

Braudy-Harris, P. (2002b) 'The subjective experience of early onset dementia: voices of the person', Unpublished paper presented at the 55th Gerontological Society of America Annual Meeting, 26 November, Boston, MA (available to download from www.dasninternational.org/).

Brijnath, B. and Manderson, L. (2008) 'Discipline in chaos: Foucault, dementia and aging in India', *Culture Medicine Psychiatry*, vol 32, pp 607-26 (DOI 10.1007/s11013-008-9111-5).

Brooker, D. (2004) 'What is person centred care for people with dementia?', *Reviews in Clinical Gerontology*, vol 13, no 3, pp 215-22.

Brooker, D. (2005) 'Dementia Care Mapping: A review of the research literature', *The Gerontologist*, vol 45, pp 11-18.

Bruce, E. and Schweitzer, P. (2008) 'Working with life history', in M. Downs and B. Bowers (eds) *Excellence in dementia care: Research into practice*, Maidenhead: McGraw-Hill/Open University Press, pp 168-186

Bruner, J. (1987) 'Life as narrative', *Social Research*, vol 54, 1, pp 11-32

Campbell, A. Gillett, G. and Jones, G. (1998) *Medical ethics* (2nd edn) Oxford: Oxford University Press.

Cantley, C. and Bowes, A. (2004) 'Dementia and social inclusion: the way forward', in A. Innes, C. Archibald and C. Murphy (eds) *Dementia and social inclusion: Marginalized groups and marginalized areas of dementia research, care and practice*, London: Jessica Kingsley Publishers, pp 255-71.

Cantley, C., Woodhouse, J. and Smith, M. (2005) *Listen to us: Involving people with dementia in planning and developing services*, Newcastle: Dementia North, Northumbria University.

Capstick, A. (2009) '"This is my turn: I'm talking now": findings and new directions from the Ex Memoria project', *Signpost: Journal of Dementia and Mental Health for Older People*, October.

Cheston, R. and Bender, M. (1999) *Understanding dementia: The man with the worried eyes*, London: Jessica Kingsley Publishers.

Clare, L., Roth, I. and Pratt, R. (2005) 'Perceptions of change over time in early-stage Alzheimer's disease: implications for understanding awareness and coping style', *Dementia: International Journal of Social Research and Practice*, vol 4, no 4, pp 487-521.

Clare, L., Rowlands, J. and Quin, R. (2008) 'Collective strength: the impact of developing a shared social identity in early-stage dementia', *Dementia*, vol 7, pp 9-30.

Clarke, P. (1996) *Deep citizenship*, Chicago, IL: Pluto Press.

Clarke, P. and Marshall, V. (2001) 'Social theory and the meaning of illness in later life: micro processes and social structure in adaptation to stroke', Paper presented at the World Congress of Gerontology, Vancouver.

Cohen, E. (2009) *Semi-citizenship in democratic politics*, Cambridge: Cambridge University Press.

Cohen, D. and Eisdorfer, C. (1986) *The Loss of Self: A family resource for the care of Alzheimer's Disease and related disorders*, London: W.W. Norton.

Corker, M. (1999) 'Differences, conflations and foundations: the limits to 'accurate' theoretical representation of disabled people's experience?', *Disability and Society*, vol 14, no 5, pp 627-42.

Corner, L. and Bond, J. (2004) 'Being at risk of dementia: fears and anxieties of older adults', *Journal of Aging Studies*, vol 18, pp 143-55.

Cotrell, V.C. and Schulz, R. (1993) 'The perspective of the patient with Alzheimer's disease: a neglected dimension of dementia research', *The Gerontologist*, vol 33, no 1, pp 205-21.

Cox, E.O. and Parsons, R.J. (1994) *Empowerment-oriented social work practice with the elderly*, Pacific Grove, CA: Brooks/Cole.

Crow, L. (1996) 'Including all of our lives: renewing the social model of disability', in C. Barnes and G. Mercer (eds) *Exploring the divide: Illness and disability*, Leeds: The Disability Press.

Czarniawska, B. (2004) *Narratives in social science research*, London: Sage Publications.

Daiute, C. and Lightfoot, C. (eds) (2004) *Narrative analysis: Studying the development of individuals in society*, Thousand Oaks, CA: Sage Publications.

Davies, S. and Nolan, M. (2008) 'Attending to relationships in dementia care', in M. Downs and B. Bowers (eds) (2008) *Excellence in dementia care: Research into practice*, Maidenhead: McGraw-Hill/Open University Press, pp 438-55.

Davis, D. (2004) 'Dementia: sociological and philosophical constructions', *Social Science and Medicine,* vol 58, no 2, pp 369-78.

Davis, J. (ed) (2002) *Stories of change: Narrative and social movements*, Albany, NY: State University of New York Press.

Dewing, J. (2002) 'From ritual to relationship: a person-centred approach to consent in qualitative research with older people who have dementia', *Dementia*, vol 1, no 2, pp 157-71.

Dewing, J. (2004) 'Concerns relating to the application of frameworks to promote personcentredness in nursing with older people', *Journal of Clinical Nursing*, vol 13, no 3a, pp 39-44.

Dewing, J. (2007) 'Participatory research, a method for process consent with persons with dementia', *Dementia*, vol 6, no 1, pp 11-25.

DH (Department of Health) (2009) *Living well with dementia: A national dementia strategy*, London: The Stationery Office.

Diamond, T. (1992) *Making gray gold: Narratives of nursing home care*, Chicago, IL: University of Chicago Press.

Downs, M. (1997) 'The emergence of the person in dementia research', *Ageing and Society*, 17, pp 597-607.

Downs, M. (2000) 'Dementia in a socio-cultural context: an idea whose time has come', *Ageing and Society,* 20, pp 369-75.

Downs, M. and Bowers, B. (eds) (2008) *Excellence in dementia care: Research into practice*, Maidenhead: McGraw-Hill/Open University Press.

Dwyer, P. (2004) *Understanding social citizenship: Themes and practices for policy and practice*, Bristol: The Policy Press.

Edvardsson, D., Winblad, B. and Sandman, P.O. (2008) 'Person-centred care for people with severe Alzheimer's disease – current status and ways forward', *The Lancet Neurology*, vol 7, pp 362-7.

Egeland, C. and Gressgard, R. (2007) 'The "will to empower": managing the complexity of the others', *Nordic Journal of Women's Studies*, vol 15, issue 4, pp 207-19.

Emirbayer, M. and Mische, A. (1998) 'What is agency?', *The American Journal of Sociology*, vol 103, no 4, pp 962-1023.

Emmel, N. (2008) *Participatory mapping: an innovative sociological method*, ESRC National Centre for Research Methods tool kit (available at http://eprints. ncrm.ac.uk/540/).

Emmel, N. and Clark, C. (2009) *The methods used in connected lives: Investigating networks, neighbourhoods and communities*, NCRM Working Paper, Swindon: National Centre for Research Methods, Economic and Social Research Council.

Estes, C., Biggs, S. and Phillipson, C. (2003) *Social policy, social theory and ageing*, Milton Keynes: Open University Press.

Faulks, K. (2000) *Citizenship*, London: Routledge.

Fontana, A. and Smith, R. (1989) 'Alzheimer's disease victims: the "unbecoming" of self and the normalization of competence', *Sociological Perspectives*, vol 32, no 1, pp 35-46.

Fook, J. (1993) *Radical casework: A theory of practice*, St. Leonard's, Australia: Allen & Unwin.

Fossey, J., Ballard, C., Juszczak, E., James, I., Alder, N., Jacoby, R. and Howard, R. (2006) 'Effect of enhanced psychosocial care on antipsychotic use in nursing home residents with severe dementia: cluster randomised trial', *British Medical Journal*, vol 332, pp 756-61.

Foucault, M. (1980) *Power/knowledge: Selected interviews and other writings, 1972-77*, Brighton: Harvester.

Foucault, M. (1988) *Madness and civilization: A history of insanity in the age of reason*, New York, NY: Vintage.

Fox, N. (1995) 'Postmodern perspectives on care: the vigil and the gift', *Critical Social Policy*, vol 15, pp 107-25.

Franssen, E.H. and Reisberg, B. (1997) 'Neurologic markers of the progression of Alzheimer's disease', *International Psychogeriatrics*, vol 9, pp 297-306.

Fratiglioni, L., Wang, H.X., Ericsson, K., Maytan, M. and Winblad, B. (2000) 'Influence of social network on occurrence of dementia: a community-based longitudinal study', *Lancet*, 355 (9212), pp 1314-19.

Freire, P. (1985) *Pedagogy of the oppressed*, New York, NY: Continuum Publishing.

French, S. (1993) 'Disability, impairment or something in between?', in J. Swain, S. French, C. Barnes and C. Thomas (eds) *Disabling barriers, enabling environments*, Buckingham: Open University Press.

Gauntlett, D. (2007) *Creative explorations: New approaches to identities and audiences*, London: Routledge.

Gillies, B. (2000) 'A memory like clockwork: accounts of living through dementia', *Aging and Mental Health*, vol 4, no 4, pp 366-74.

Gould, C. (1988) *Rethinking democracy: Freedom and social cooperation in politics, economy and society*, Cambridge: Cambridge University Press.

Graham, R. (2004) 'Cognitive citizenship: access to hip surgery for people with dementia', *Health*, vol 8, no 3, pp 295-310.

Hachinski, V. (2008) 'Shifts in thinking about dementia' *Journal of American Medical Association*, 12, 300, (18), pp 2172-3.

Hamer, S. and Collinson, G. (2005) *Achieving evidence-based practice*, London: Bailliere Tindall.

Harding, N. and Palfry, N. (1997) *The social construction of dementia: Confused professionals?*, London: Jessica Kingsley Publishers.

Harris, P.B. and Sterin, G.J. (1999) 'Insider's perspective: defining and preserving the self in dementia', *Journal of Mental Health and Aging*, vol 5, pp 241-56.

Harrison, C. (1993) 'Personhood, dementia and the integrity of life', *Canadian Journal on Aging*, vol 12, no 4, pp 428-40.

Health Advisory Service (1983) *The rising tide: Developing services for mental illness in old age*, Sutton: Health Advisory Service.

Health Development Agency (2004) *Developing healthier communities: An introductory course for people using community development approaches to improve health and tackle health inequalities*, London: Health Development Agency.

Heater, D. (1999) *What is citizenship?*, Malden: Blackwell Publishers.

Heater, D. (2004) *Citizenship: The civic ideal in world history, politics and education*, London: Longman.

Henderson, D. (1995) 'Consciousness raising in participatory research: method and methodology for emancipatory nursing inquiry', *Advanced Nursing Science*, vol 17, no 3, pp 58-69.

Henderson, J.N and Traphagan, J.W. (2005) 'Cultural factors in dementia: perspectives from the anthropology of aging', *Alzheimer Disease and Associated Disorders* vol 19, no 4, pp 272-4.

Herskovits, E. (1995) 'Struggling over subjectivity: debates about the "self" and Alzheimer's disease', *Medical Anthropology Quarterly*, vol 9, no 2, pp 146-64.

Hirschman, K.B., Joyce, C.M., James, B.D., Xie, S.X. and Karlawish, J.H.T. (2005) 'Do Alzheimer's Disease patients want to participate in a treatment decision, and would their caregivers let them?', *Gerontologist*, vol 45, no 3, pp 381-8.

Hockey, J. and James, A. (2003) *Social identities across the life course*, London: Palgrave Macmillan.

Holmes, C. and Wilkinson, D. (2000) 'Molecular biology of Alzheimer's disease', *Advances in Psychiatric Treatment*, vol 6, pp 193-200.

Hughes, B. and Paterson, K. (1997) 'The social model of disability and the disappearing body: towards a sociology of impairment', *Disability & Society*, vol 12, no 3, pp 325-40.

Hulko, W. (2002) 'Making the links: social theories, experiences of people with dementia, and intersectionality', in A. Leibing and L. Scheinkman (eds) *The diversity of Alzheimer's disease: Different approaches and contexts*, Rio de Janeiro: CUCA-IPUB, pp 231-64.

Hulko, W. (2005) 'From doctor to "silly patient": seeing beyond the disease label', *International Journal of Epidemiology*, vol 34, no 1, pp 36-9.

Hulko, W. (2009) 'From "not a big deal" to "hellish": experiences of older people with dementia', *Journal of Aging Studies*, vol 24, no 1, pp 44-55.

Humphrey, J. (1999) 'Disabled people and the politics of difference', *Disability and Society*, vol 14, no 2, pp 173-88.

Ignatieff, M. (1989) 'Citizenship and moral narcissism', *The Political Quarterly*, vol 60, pp 63-74.

Ineichen, B. (1987) 'Measuring the rising tide: how many dementia cases will there be in 2001?', *British Journal of Psychiatry*, 150, pp 195-200.

Innes, A. (2002) 'The social and political context of formal dementia care provision', *Ageing and Society*, 22, pp 483-499.

Innes, A. (2009) *Dementia studies*, London: Sage Publications.

Innes, A., Archibald, C. and Murphy, C. (eds) (2004) *Dementia and social inclusion: Marginalised groups and marginalised areas of dementia research, care and practice*, London: Jessica Kingsley Publishers.

Isin, E. and Nielsen, G. (2008) *Acts of citizenship*, London: Zed Books.

Isin, E. and Wood, P. (eds) (1999) *Citizenship and identity*, London: Sage Publications.

Jackson, L. (2009) 'Living positively with a diagnosis of dementia', 17 February, Alzheimer Society British Columbia (www.thememorybank.ca/node/152).

Judd, S. (2007) 'Citizenship and dementia', *The Journal of Dementia Care*, vol 15, no 3, pp 19-21.

Keady, J., Williams, S. and Hughes-Roberts, J. (2005) 'Emancipatory practice development through life-story work: changing care in a memory clinic in North Wales', *Practice Development in Health Care*, vol 4, no 4, pp 203-12.

Kelly, M. (1993) *Designing for people with dementia in the context of the building standards*, Dementia Services Development Centre, Stirling.

Killick, J. and Allan, K. (2001) *Communication and the care of people with dementia*, Buckingham: Open University Press.

King's Fund Centre (1986) *Living well into old age: Applying principles of good practice to services for people with dementia. Report Number 63.* London: King's Fund Publishing Office.

Kitchin, R. (1998) 'Out of place, "knowing one's place": space, power and the exclusion of disabled people', *Disability and Society*, vol 13, no 3, pp 343-56.

Kittay, E. F. (1999) 'Welfare, dependency and a public ethic of care', in G. Mink (ed) *Whose welfare?*, New York, NY: Cornell University Press, 1999, pp.189-213.

Kitwood, T. (1990) 'The dialectics of dementia: with particular reference to Alzheimer's disease', *Ageing and Society*, vol 10, pp 177-96.

Kitwood, T. (1992) 'Towards a theory of dementia care: personhood and well-being', *Ageing and Society*, vol 12, no 3, pp 269-87.

Kitwood, T. (1993) 'Frames of reference for an understanding of dementia', in J. Johnson and R. Slater (1993) (eds) *Ageing and later life*, Buckingham: Open University Press, pp 100-106.

Kitwood, T. (1997a) *Dementia reconsidered: The person comes first*, Buckingham: Open University Press.

Kitwood, T. (1997b) 'The experience of dementia', *Ageing and Mental Health*, vol 1, no 1, pp 13-22.

Kontos, P. (2004) 'Ethnographic reflections on selfhood, embodiment and Alzheimer's disease', *Aging & Society*, vol 24, pp 829-49.

Kontos, P. (2005) 'Embodied selfhood in Alzheimer's disease: rethinking person centred dementia care', *Dementia: International Journal of Social Research and Practice*, vol 4, no 4, pp 553-70.

Kvale, S. (1996) *InterViews: An introduction to qualitative research interviewing*, Thousand Oaks, CA: Sage Publications.

Langdon, S., Eagle, A. and Warner, J. (2007) 'Making sense of dementia in the social world', *Social Science and Medicine*, vol 64, no 4, pp 989-1000.

Link, B.G. and Phelan, J.C. (2006) 'Stigma and its public health implications', *The Lancet,* 367, pp 528-9.

Lister, R. (2003) *Citizenship: Feminist perspectives,* London: Macmillan.

Lister, R. (2007) 'Inclusive citizenship: realizing the potential', *Citizenship Studies,* vol 11, no 1, pp 49-61.

Lyman, K. (1998) 'Living with Alzheimer's disease: the creation of meaning among persons with dementia', *Journal of Clinical Ethics,* vol 9, no 1, pp 49-57.

McCall, L. (2005) 'The complexity of intersectionality', *Signs: Journal of Women in Culture and Society,* vol 30, no 3, pp 1771-800.

McColgan, G. (2005) 'A place to sit: resistance strategies used to create privacy and home by people with dementia', *Journal of Contemporary Ethnography,* vol 34, no 4, pp 410-33.

McKillop, J. and Wilkinson, H. (2004) 'Make it easy on yourself! Advice to researchers from someone with dementia on being interviewed', *Dementia,* vol 3, no 2, pp 117-25.

Makin, T. (1995) 'The social model of disability', *Counselling,* November, p 274.

Marks, D. (1999) *Disability: Controversial debates and psychosocial perspectives,* London: Routledge.

Marshall, M. (2001) 'Care settings and care environments', in C. Cantley (ed) *A handbook of dementia care,* Buckingham: Open University Press, pp 173-86.

Marshall, T.H. (1949/92) 'Citizenship and social class', in T.H. Marshall and T. Bottomore, *Citizenship and social class,* London: Pluto Press, pp 3-51.

Martin, G. and Younger, D. (2000) 'Anti-oppressive practice: a route to the empowerment of people with dementia through communication and choice', *Journal of Psychiatric and Mental Health Nursing,* vol 7, pp 59-67.

Mason, J. and Davies, K. (2009) Coming to our senses? A critical approach to sensory methodology. NCRM Working Paper. Realities, Morgan Centre, Manchester, UK. (Unpublished) (available to download from http://eprints. ncrm.ac.uk/538/).

Miesen, B. (2006) 'Attachment in dementia: bound from birth?', in B. Miesen and G. Jones (eds) *Care-giving in dementia: Research and applications,* London: Routledge, pp 105-32.

Mitchell, R. (2005) *Captured memories: A photography project in a drop-in centre,* Stirling: Dementia Services Development Centre.

MIND (1999) *Creating accepting communities: Report of the Mind Inquiry into Social Exclusion,* London: Mind Publications.

Mitnitski, A.B., Graham, J.E., Mogilner, A.J. and Rockwood, K. (1999) 'The rate of decline in functions in Alzheimer's disease and other dementias', *Journal of Gerontology: Medical Sciences,* vol 54, no 2, pp M65-9.

Moore, M., Beazley, S. and Maelzer, J. (1998) *Researching disability issues,* Buckingham: Open University Press.

Morris, J. (1997) 'Care or empowerment? A disability rights perspective', *Social Policy and Administration,* vol 31, no 1, pp 54-60.

MRC-CFAS Neuropathology Group (2001) 'Pathological correlates of late-onset dementia in a multicentre, community-based population in England and Wales, Neuropathology Group of the Medical Research Council Cognitive Function and Ageing Study (MRC-CFAS)', *Lancet*, vol 357, no 9251, pp 169-75.

Mullaly, R. (2007) *The new structural social work*, Ontario: Oxford University Press

Murphy, J., Gray, C. and Cox, C. (2007) 'The use of talking mats to improve communication and quality of care for people with dementia', *Housing, Care and Support*, vol 10, no 3, pp 21-5.

Nagahata, K., Fukushima, T., Ishibashi, N., Takahashi, Y. and Moriyama, M. (2004) 'A Soundscape Study: What kinds of sounds can elderly people affected by dementia recollect?', *Noise & Health*, vol 6, no 24, pp 63-73.

Nolan, M., Ryan, T., Enderby, P. and Reid, D. (2002) 'Towards a more inclusive vision of dementia care and research', *Dementia: International Journal of Social Research and Practice*, vol 2, pp 193-211.

Nolan, M., Brown, R., Davies, S., Nolan, J and Keady, J. (2006) *The Senses Framework: Improving Care for Older People Through a Relationship-Centred Approach. Getting Research into Practice (GRiP)* Report No 2, University of Sheffield.

Nuffield Council on Bioethics (2009) *Dementia: Ethical issues*, London: Nuffield Council on Bioethics.

O'Connor, D. (1995) 'Supporting spousal caregivers: exploring the meaning of service use', *Families in Society*, vol 76, no 5, pp 296-305.

O'Connor, D. (1999) 'Living with a memory-impaired spouse: (Re) cognizing the experience', *Canadian Journal of Aging*, vol 18, no 2, pp 211-35.

O'Connor, D. (2002) 'Toward empowerment: ReVisioning family support groups', *Social Work with Groups*, vol 25, no 4, pp 37-56.

O'Connor, D., Phinney, A., Smith, A., Small, J., Purves, B., Perry, J., Drance, E., Donnelly, M., Chaudhury, H. and Beattie, L. (2007) 'Personhood in dementia care: developing a research agenda for broadening the vision', *Dementia: International Journal of Social Research and Practice*, vol 6, no 1, pp 121-42.

O'Connor, D., Phinney, A. and Hulko, W. (2009) 'Dementia at the intersections: a unique case study exploring social location', *Journal of Aging Studies*, vol 24, no 1, pp 30-9.

O'Connor, D., Chan, S.M., Hulko, W., Stern, L., and Yan, M. (forthcoming) 'Contextualizing dementia: conceptualizing culture', *Dementia: International Journal of Social Research and Practice*.

Oliver, M. (1996) *Understanding disability: From theory to practice*, London: Macmillan Press.

Opie, A. (2000) *Thinking teams, thinking clients: Knowledge-based teamwork*, New York, NY: Columbia University Press.

Pakulski, J. (1997) 'Cultural citizenship', *Citizenship Studies*, vol 1, no 1, pp 73-86.

Paré, A. (2002) 'Keeping writing in its place: a participatory action approach to workplace communication', in B. Mirel and R. Spilka (ed) *Reshaping technical communication: New directions and challenges for the 21st century*, Mahwah, NJ: Lawrence Erlbaum, pp 57-80.

Parker, J. (2001) 'Interrogating person-centered dementia care in social work and social care', *Journal of Social Work*, vol 1, no 3, pp 329-45.

Paterson, K. and Hughes, B. (1999) 'Disability studies and phenomenology: the carnal politics of everyday life', *Disability and Society*, vol 14, no 5, pp 597-610.

Pattie, C., Seyd, P. and Whiteley, P. (2004) *Citizenship in Britain: Values, participation and democracy*, Cambridge: Cambridge University Press.

Phinney, A. (2008) 'Towards understanding subjective experience of dementia', in M. Downs and B. Bowers (eds) *Excellence in dementia care: Research into practice*, Maidenhead: McGraw Hill/Open University Press, pp 35-51.

Phinney, A. and Chesla, C. A. (2003) 'The lived body in dementia', *Journal of Aging Studies*, 17, pp 283-99.

Phoenix, C., Smith, B. and Sparkes, A. (2010) 'Narrative analysis in aging studies: a typology for consideration', *Journal of Aging Studies*, vol 24, pp 1-11.

Pink, S. (2007) *Doing visual ethnography* (2nd edn), London: Sage Publications.

Pink, S. (2009) *Doing sensory ethnography*, London: Sage Publications.

Pointon, B. (2007) 'Reflections on making a health complaint and the health ombudsman's findings on the care of Malcolm Pointon' (www.alzheimers.org. uk/News_and_Campaigns/Campaigning/PDF/ombudsman_pointon.pdf).

Popper, K. (1999) *The logic of scientific discovery*, London and New York, NY: Routledge.

Post, S. (2000) *The moral challenge of Alzheimer's disease: Ethical issues from diagnosis to dying*, Baltimore, MD: Johns Hopkins University.

Pratt, R. (2002) 'Nobody's ever asked how I felt', in H. Wilkinson (ed) *The perspectives of people with dementia: Research methods and motivations*, London: Jessica Kingsley Publishers, pp 25-46.

Priestley, M. (2004) 'Generating debates: why we need a life course approach to disability issues', in J. Swain, S. French, C. Barnes and C. Thomas (eds) *Disabling barriers, enabling environments*, London, SAGE, pp 94-99.

Prior, D., Stewart, J. and Walsh, K. (1995) *Citizenship: Rights and community participation*, London: Pitman.

Proctor, G. (2001) 'Listening to older women with dementia: relationships, voices and power', *Disability and Society*, vol 16, no 3, pp 361-76.

Ray, R. E. (2000) *Beyond nostalgia: Aging and life-story writing*, Charlottesville, VA: University Press of Virginia.

Reason, P. (ed) (1994) *Participation in human inquiry*, London: Sage Publications.

Rewston, C. and Moniz-Cook, E. (2008) Understanding and alleviating emotional distress, in M. Downs and B. Bowers (eds) (2008) *Excellence in dementia care: Research into practice*, Maidenhead: McGraw-Hill/Open University Press, pp 249-63.

Roberts, G. (2000) 'Narrative and severe mental illness: what places do stories have in an evidence based world', *Advances in Psychiatric Treatment*, vol 6, pp 432-41.

Robinson, E. (2002) 'Should people with Alzheimer's disease take part in research?', in H. Wilkinson (ed) *The perspective of people with dementia: Research methods and motivations*, London: Jessica Kingsley Publishers, pp 9-24.

Rosenwald, G.C. and Ochberg, R.L. (1992) *Storied lives: The cultural politics of self-understanding*, New Haven, CT: Yale University Press.

Rossiter, A. (2000) The postmodern feminist condition: new conditions for social work, in B. Fawcett, B. Featherstone, J. Fook and A. Rossiter (eds), *Practice and research in social work: Postmodern feminist perspectives*, Abingdon: Routledge, pp 24-38.

Roulstone, A. and Barnes, C. (eds) (2005) *Working futures: Disabled people, policy and social inclusion*, Bristol: The Policy Press.

Rundqvist, E.M. and Severinsson, E.I. (1999) 'Caring relationships with patients suffering from dementia – an interview study', *Journal of Advanced Nursing*, vol 29, no 4, pp 800-7.

Ryan, T., Nolan, M., Reid, D. and Enderby, P (2008) 'Using the senses framework to achieve relationship-centred dementia care services', *Dementia: International journal of social research and practice*, vol 7, no 1, pp 71-93.

Sabat, S. (2001) *The experiences of Alzheimer's disease: Life through a tangled veil*, Oxford: Blackwell Publishers.

Sabat, S. (2002) 'Surviving manifestations of selfhood in Alzheimer's disease: a case study', *Dementia: International Journal of Social Research and Practice*, vol 1, no 1, pp 25-36.

Sabat, S. (2003) 'Some potential benefits of creating research partnerships with people with Alzheimer's disease', *Research Policy and Planning*, vol 21, no 2, pp 5-12.

Sabat, S. (2005) 'Capacity for decision-making in Alzheimer's disease: selfhood, positioning and semiotic persons', *Australian and New Zealand Journal of Psychiatry*, 39, pp 1030-5.

Sabat, S. and Harre, R. (1992) 'The construction and deconstruction of self in Alzheimer's disease', *Ageing and Society*, vol 12, pp 443-61.

Sayce, L. (2000) *From psychiatric patient to citizen: Overcoming discrimination and exclusion*, London: Macmillan Press Ltd.

Scourfield, P. (2007) 'Helping older people in residential care remain full citizens', *British Journal of Social Work*, vol 37, pp 1135-52.

SDWG (Scottish Dementia Working Group) (2007) *SDWG 2007/8 report: A year of progress and achievement* (www.sdwg.org.uk/talks-and-publications/).

Seddon, D., Lang, R. and Daines, V. (2001) 'Mainstreaming disability issues into development studies – in theory and practice', Paper presented at the 14th annual meeting of the Disability Studies Association, Winnipeg, Canada.

Sherwin, S. (1992) *No longer patient: Feminist ethics and health care*, Philadelphia, PA: Temple University Press.

Shilling, C. (1997) 'The undersocialised conception of the embodied agent in modern sociology', *Sociology*, vol 31, no 4, pp 737-54.

Shotter, J. (1993) 'Psychology and citizenship: identity and belonging', in B. Turner (ed) *Citizenship and social theory*, London: Sage Publications, pp 115-38.

Silver, C. (2008) 'Participatory approaches to social research', in N. Gilbert *Researching social life* (3rd edn), London: Sage Publications, pp 101-24.

Skeggs, B. (2004) *Class, self, culture*, London: Routledge.

Sloane, P., Brooker, D., Cohen, L., Douglass, C., Edelman, P., Fulton, B., Jarrott, S., Kasayka, R., Kuhn, D., Preisser, J., Williams, C. and Zimmerman, S. (2007) 'Dementia care mapping as a research tool', *International Journal of Geriatric Psychiatry*, vol 22, pp 580-9.

Smith, A. (2009) Decision-making as social practice: exploring the relevance of Bourdieu's concepts of habitus and symbolic capital', in D. O'Connor and B. Purves (eds) (2009) *Decision-making, personhood and dementia: Exploring the interface*, London: Jessica Kingsley Publishers, pp 37-46.

Smith, D. (2005) *Institutional ethnography: A sociology for people*, Oxford: AltaMira Press.

Social Exclusion Unit (2006) *Sure start to later life: Ending inequalities for older people*, London: Office of the Deputy Prime Minister.

Stone, E. and Priestley, M. (1996) 'Parasites, pawns and partners: disability research and the role of non-disabled researchers', *British Journal of Sociology*, vol 47, no 4, p 109.

Surr, C. (2006) 'Preservation of self in people with dementia living in residential care: a socio-biographical approach', *Social Science and Medicine*, vol 62, no 7, pp 1720-30.

Swain, J. and French, S. (1998) 'Normality and disabling care', in A. Brechin et al (eds) (1998) *Care Matters: concepts, practice and research in health and social care*, London: Sage Publications.

Swain, J., French, S. and Cameron, C. (2003) *Controversial issues in a disabling society*, Buckingham: Open University Press.

Sweeting, H. and Gilhooly, M. (1997) 'Dementia and the phenomenon of social death', *Sociology of Health and Illness*, vol 19, pp 93-117.

Taylor, B.D. and Tripodes, S. (2001) 'The effects of driving cessation on the elderly with dementia and their caregivers', *Accident Analysis and Prevention*, vol 33, pp 519-28.

Taylor, R. (2009) *Alzheimer's from the inside out*, July, issue 17 (www.richardtaylorphd. com/newsletters/).

Thake, S. (2008) *Individualism and consumerism: Reframing the debate*, York: Joseph Rowntree Foundation.

Thomas, P. (2004) Personal email correspondence, Thursday, 29 April.

Trachtenerg, D. and Trojanowski, J. (2008) 'Dementia: a word to be forgotten', *Archives of Neurology*, vol 65, no 5, pp 593-5.

Trivedi, P. and Wykes, T. (2002) 'From passive subjects to equal partners: qualitative review of user involvement in research', *British Journal of Psychiatry*, vol 181, pp 468-72.

Tsai, D. (2009) A Confucian two-dimensional approach to personhood, dementia, and decision making, in D. O'Connor and B. Purves (eds) (2009) *Decision-making, personhood and dementia: Exploring the interface*, London: Jessica Kingsley Publishers, pp 58-69.

Turner, B. (1990) 'Outline of a theory of citizenship', *Sociology*, vol 24, no 2, pp 189-217.

Turner, B. (1986) *Citizenship and capitalism: The debate over reformism*, London: Allen and Unwin.

UN (United Nations) Programme on Ageing and the International Association of Gerontology (2007) *Research agenda on aging for the 21st century* (www.un.org/ageing/researchagenda.html).

Vodde, R. and Gallant, J.P. (2002) 'Bridging the gap between micro and macro practice: large scale change and a unified model of narrative-deconstructive practice', *Journal of Social Work Education*, vol 38, no 3, pp 439-58.

Walker, A. (1999) 'Older people and health services: the challenge of empowerment', in M. Purdy and D. Banks (eds), *Health and exclusion: Policy and practice in health provision*, London: Routledge, pp 159-77.

Walton, J. (1999) 'Young-onset dementia', in T. Adams and C. Clarke (eds) (1999) *Dementia care: Developing partnerships in practice*, London: Balliere Tindall, pp 257-80.

Warren, C. and Karner, T. (2005) *Discovering qualitative methods: Field research, interviews, and analysis*, Los Angeles, CA: Roxbury Press.

Weedon, C. (1987) *Feminist practice and poststructuralist theory*, Oxford: Basil Blackwell.

Wenger, G., Scott, A. and Seddon, S. (2002) 'The experience of caring for older people with dementia in rural areas: using services', *Ageing and Mental Health*, vol 6, no 1, pp 30-8.

White, M. and Epston, D. (1990) *Narrative means to therapeutic ends*, New York, NY: W.W. Norton & Co Ltd.

Whitlatch, C.J., Feinberg, L.F. and Tucke, S.S. (2005) 'Measuring the values and preferences for everyday care of persons with cognitive impairment and their family caregivers', *The Gerontologist*, vol 45, pp 370-80.

Widdicombe, S. (1993) 'Autobiography and change: rhetoric and authenticity of gothic style', in E. Burman and I. Parker (eds) *Discourse analytic research*, New York: Routledge, pp 106-27.

Wilkinson, H. (2002) 'Including people with dementia in research: methods and motivations', in H. Wilkinson (ed) *The perspectives of people with dementia: Research methods and motivations*, London: Jessica Kingsley Publishers, pp 9-25.

Williams, S. and Keady, J. (2006) 'Editorial: the narrative voice of people with dementia', *Dementia: International Journal of Social Research and Practice*, vol 5, no 2, pp 163-6.

Wislowski, A. (2006) 'Voting rights for older Americans with dementia: implications for health care providers', *Nursing Outlook*, vol 54, pp 68-73.

Woods, R. (2001) 'Discovering the person with Alzheimer's disease: cognitive, emotional and behavioural aspects' *Aging and Mental Health*, 5 (supplement 1), S7-16.

Index

Note: Page numbers followed by *fig* or *tab* refer to information in a figure or a table respectively.